W9-AQT-449

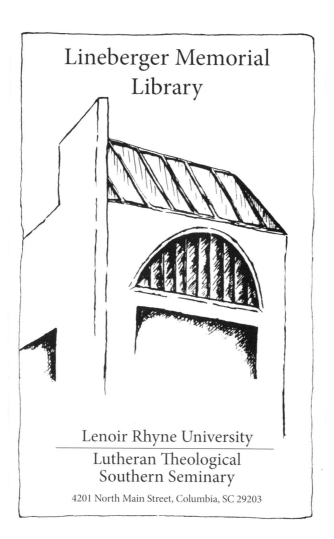

Lineberger Memorial
Library

Lenoir Rhyne University

Lutheran Theological
Southern Seminary

4201 North Main Street, Columbia, SC 29203

WAR AND REDEMPTION

"... Nation shall not lift up sword against nation, neither shall they learn war anymore."

Isaiah

The hope of all those who have tasted the bitter reality of war.

War and Redemption

Treatment and Recovery in Combat-related
Posttraumatic Stress Disorder

LARRY DEWEY

ASHGATE

© Larry Dewey 2004

All rights reserved. No part of this publication may be reproduced, stored in a retrieval system, or transmitted in any form or by any means, electronic, mechanical, photocopying, recording, or otherwise without the prior permission of the publisher.

Larry Dewey has asserted his right under the Copyright, Designs and Patents Act, 1988, to be identified as the author of this work.

Published by
Ashgate Publishing Limited
Wey Court East
Union Road
Farnham
Surrey, GU9 7PT
England

Ashgate Publishing Company
Suite 420
101 Cherry Street
Burlington,
VT 05401-4405
USA

Ashgate website: http://www.ashgate.com

British Library Cataloguing in Publication Data
Dewey, Larry
    War and redemption : treatment and recovery in
    combat-related posttraumatic stress disorder
    1.Posttraumatic stress disorder - Treatment 2.War neuroses
    3.Veterans - Mental health 4.War - Psychological aspects
    I. Title
    616.8'521206

Library of Congress Cataloging-in-Publication Data
Dewey, Larry.
    War and redemption : treatment and recovery in combat-related posttraumatic stress
    disorder / Larry Dewey.
        p. cm.
    Includes bibliographical references and index.
    ISBN 0-7546-4165-1
        1.Posttraumatic stress disorder. 2.Veterans--Mental health. I.Title.

    RC552.P67D495 2004
    616.85'21–dc22
                                                          2003062887
ISBN 13: 978 0 7546 4165 0

Reprinted 2006, 2008, 2012

Typeset in Times New Roman by SetSystems Ltd, Saffron Walden, Essex.

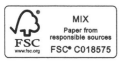

Printed and bound in Great Britain by the
MPG Books Group, UK

Contents

List of Figures

Acknowledgements

Karen Cooke and Nadeyne Maurer provided valuable guidance in using the computer. John Mangan made the pictures possible. Wayne Tippets gave me time I would not otherwise have had. Mark Heilman, Patrick Costello and Bill Pittman were always listening and supporting. Maggie Morris encouraged me for almost two decades. James Branahl, James Dewey and Gary Richardson critiqued the manuscript with fresh eyes. Thomas Draper gave essential, detailed criticism and advice. Johan Verhulst helped me make a critical connection. Erik Fisher patiently praised, challenged and corrected until it was a much better work. Teresa Dewey never tired of making me a better writer. She has spent years doing it. This book became a reality only through her constant help.

Jacket cover: Multimedia painting of Vietcong AK-47 used with permission of Myke Knutson.

Passages from Brendan Phibbs' *The Other Side of Time* used with permission.

Figures 2.1 and 2.2 used with permission of the painter Myke Knutson.

Figures 2.3, 2.4, 2.5, 2.8 courtesy of the US Library of Congress.

Figures 2.6, 2.7, 2.9, 2.10 courtesy of the US National Archives.

Figure 2.11 *Marines Call It That 2000 Yard Stare*. Courtesy of the National Museum of the US Army.

Poem *The Group* used with permission of the author Dan Koper.

Poems *The Warrior* and *Man from Another World* used with permission of the author.

Introduction

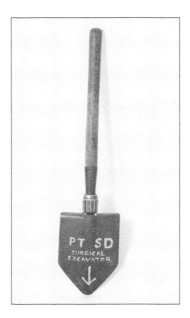

Figure 0.1   Walt's pack shovel

Pictured above is a World War II pack shovel given to me by one of my combat vets, Walt, as he was terminating group therapy. He painted the inscription on the back of the shovel: "PTSD SURGICAL EXCAVATOR." He and the group joked that it was what I did for a living. He wanted me to have the shovel because it had saved his life more times than anything else in Italy. Digging deep was often the only way to survive German artillery. He felt that, in the same way, our "digging deep" into his war-related emotional trauma had saved him emotionally. When he presented it to me in group, the other men concurred. I have been educated and changed by digging deep into war trauma with my veteran patients. I hope to share with the reader what my patients and other veterans in their personal writings have taught me about the pain of good men who fight, kill and survive war. I also want to share the remarkable story of their coping, recovery and redemptive healing.

I never anticipated the power of what these veterans have taught me. We will explore the dark side first – the pain, horror and burden of war and killing. Then we will turn to the remarkable things they have taught me about recovering from life's worst traumas. I hope to show you in their own stories and words what they have painfully led me to appreciate over the last 20 years.

Many years ago I read Audie Murphy's autobiography *To Hell and Back*. It chronicles his experiences as a rifleman in WWII. His title succinctly sums up what war is about for those who fight it. It is a journey to Hell: physically, emotionally and spiritually. Men who have made this journey are reluctant to discuss it. They are slow to share the truth about their war experiences with anyone who did not accompany them. They share their most painful and traumatic experiences only with those they trust.

When I was in my psychiatry residency at Yale Medical School, one of my psychotherapy supervisors, Charlie Gardner, taught me a lesson that has been crucial in my successful work with vets. For several months Dr. Gardner had been seeing a young man at the Yale Psychiatric Institute, a long-term treatment facility specializing in the care of the most seriously ill. Initially they seemed to be making very little progress together. Abruptly the therapy began moving forward. After three or four months of rapid progress with this young man, Dr. Gardner commented in a therapy session on this abrupt change for the better and wondered what the patient thought had brought this about. The patient, who was being treated for his first psychotic break, responded, according to Dr. Gardner, as follows:

I was looking out the window of the Institute, lost in thought. It was raining heavily. I saw an old Volkswagen Beetle drive in and park. A man jumped out in the rain and dashed for the door of the institute, trying to avoid getting soaked. It made me laugh. Then I realized that you were that man, and that you had been coming to see me weekly for months. I decided then that I could trust you. That is when we started making progress.

Dr. Gardner's point was not lost on me. I recognized that for many clients, therapists have to be very patient, constant and quietly persistent before trust can develop. We have to prove we are reliable and will be available to help them for as long as they need us. Since effective therapy usually depends on the patient sharing some of his or her most troubling experiences, thoughts and feelings with his clinician, little effective treatment can occur without trust.

One of the reasons my veteran patients have shared with me the material that made this book worth writing is that I have been here for them for over two decades. They see me as a reliable, trustworthy and calm listener. Many times I have seen a man for years before he shares what has troubled him most. Often I am told, "This is the first time I have shared this with anyone." They have shared with me what war and their recovery from war has been like for them. They have taught me things about war trauma and its treatment that I couldn't have learned from any other source, unless I had lived through it with them.[1]

As a rule there are two large groups of combatants: those who fight on the ground in a more or less face-to-face battle with the enemy, and those who fight from planes and ships and experience a different set of horrors. In this book we will explore the experiences of both.

Out of the hundreds of combat vets I have treated over the last 20 years, I selected case material, thoughts and experiences from 65 to use in this book. I felt these were representative of the larger body of men I have treated. They include two who served in tanks, three artillerymen, three helicopter pilots or crewmen, three from the airborne forces, four medics or corpsmen, six from Special Forces or SOG – the US Army's Special Operations Group (two of which were USAF air commandos working with SOG), six who flew in bombers, nine seamen and 33 Marine Corps riflemen or US Army infantrymen. Four served in multiple combat roles. Four were prisoners of war. Forty-one served in WWII, eight in Korea, 17 in Vietnam (four in multiple wars) and one in Desert Storm.

I use quotes liberally in this book, especially in relating what combatants have told me about themselves and their experiences. These are not taken from recordings, but I have shown what I wrote to 44 of those I have quoted, and they have corrected and authorized what I have said. Often we spent many hours together editing their stories, which are now as accurate as their memories, diaries and other notes allow. Except where requested by the veteran, I have used fictitious names. These 44 comprise almost all the major cases I use. For others who are now dead, my memory and personal notes with all their weaknesses are all I have. In a few cases I can no longer locate men I discuss. In these few cases, as with the deceased, I have withheld details that might have allowed identification of the veteran. Many of the stories quoted are compilations of what a man may have told me over many sessions and group meetings rather than in one sitting. Some crucial details of a particular event might not have been shared with me until years after most of the story was told.

The process of presenting these stories to the veterans I treat has been very enlightening for me and therapeutic for them. As we worked on the book together and they read the chapter or chapters that contained what I had written about them, I realized that a book I initially thought I was writing for therapists was also being written for combat veterans, their families and anyone else who wants to know what war and recovery from war are truly like. My veterans constantly remarked to me how helpful it was to read those chapters and how they hoped to read more. This often led to further significant gains in therapy. They also wished to have their families read the book so they could understand the things the veteran had been through, but which they had never been able to share.

In this book I refer to the vet as "he" because I have not yet personally treated any women who fought in combat. As the military is changing, I suspect I will treat female combatants before I have finished my work for the VA. I have had the privilege of working with nurses and other non-combat medical personnel who served during wartime. They have their own burden of grief and pain from caring for the wounded and dying that are the sad harvest of war.

Combat vets start out as a cross section of normal humans. The men described here are regular guys in every respect, except for experiencing combat. I see in them all the ordinary weaknesses, problems and strengths of humanity. Although their combat experiences may have left them with physical, emotional and spiritual challenges and symptoms, most of them are stronger in the end because they have faced these challenges and prevailed.

I suggest that some combat vets consider reading this book starting with Chapter 5 or Chapter 6. They do not need to descend into hell again in their own minds by reading Chapters 1 to 4. I believe they will benefit more by reading the therapy chapters first and then returning to the beginning chapters after reading to Chapter 17.

Note

1   Several years ago I read a science fiction novel that aptly described part of my work. On a distant planet inhabited by humans, a technology had been developed that allowed people to record an accurate and detailed record of the experiences of their lives,

including their emotions and thoughts. These "life records" were stored in a vast archive called the "Library of Souls." Those with proper clearance and legitimate reasons were allowed to use this library. To do so they would sit in a special seat, put on a headset, attach the appropriate electrodes to their heads and start playing the recording. They would then experience the full impact of the person's life as if they were living it. All this would occur at the speed of thought. It allowed them to learn from others' lives the things they had learned from their experiences, without having to live those lives themselves. In many ways my vets have painstakingly done this for me.

Silverberg, Robert, *The Majipoor Chronicles*, New York: Arbor House, 1981. Bantam, 1983.

Part I

The Descent into Hell

In this section of the book we explore the deep pain and burden of killing. We explore the role of propaganda in starting the killing of war and the role love plays in helping combatants wage war to its end. I portray through my patients' stories what the personal war of the ordinary combatant is like and the burden of guilt, grief and pain he often carries afterwards. I present the deeper misery of killing civilians and other friendly combatants. Finally we look at the forces that cause men to break down in war and afterwards: overwhelming grief, exhaustion, guilt and fear, in that relative order. We finish by clarifying some of the misconceptions that have arisen over the role of fear in combat breakdown and in prolonging the combatant's suffering through the rest of his life.

Chapter 1

The Burden of Killing

Ed had just turned 18 and had been married to his childhood sweetheart about two months when he joined the US Army in late 1943. He came from a rural community in Idaho and ended up in the 10th Mountain Division. A lot of young men from the West were put in the same unit. They trained hard to fight in rough terrain and on skis. Ed was small and wiry. He was an excellent shot and became a scout.

In late 1944 they were shipped to Italy. On the boat over he was pissing in the ship's head when two unfamiliar, burly men from the division entered. They teased him about his youthful appearance: "What are you, our water boy? I thought we only enlisted men in this outfit!"

After arriving in Italy, they were moving across an open field toward the front lines when they were caught in their first artillery barrage. Ed noticed ahead of him a group of men standing around a wounded man. He ran to them and yelled at them to run for the cover of the trees. The casualty had lost his foot at the ankle. Ed applied a tourniquet and called the medics. As they were carrying him off, the wounded man recognized Ed from the encounter at sea and whispered, "Why, if it isn't the little runt from the ship's head saving my life."

The division moved into intense combat in the mountains of Italy. They remained locked in combat with the Germans until the end of the war. On a scouting patrol Ed found an unfamiliar infantryman from the division who had obviously been abandoned in a previous firefight. Eviscerated by a large caliber shell, his entrails were grotesquely exposed. In a hoarse whisper he begged, "Please, please, please kill me." Having nothing else to offer, and knowing the soldier was mortally wounded, Ed put his hands over the soldier's mouth and nose and suffocated him to relieve his pain. When we first began working together 40 years later, this "snuffing out a life with my bare hands" still troubled him.

A few weeks later Ed's company was trying to drive the Germans from a stone farmhouse. Ed was laying down covering fire on the door. At a movement in the doorway he fired. The momentum of the fleeing Italian child carried him out the door. The Germans were flanked and retreated in time for Ed to hold the child he had shot in his arms as the child died. The question, "How can I be forgiven for killing an innocent boy?" was still painfully gnawing at Ed's soul many years later.

As a company scout, Ed was often sent on dangerous patrols. On one night patrol he was captured by two German sentries. They disarmed him and took him to a nearby woodshed, where he became convinced they were going to rape and torture him. One went outside for a moment to relieve himself. Ed had noticed a small ax in one corner. The second soldier's inattention allowed Ed just enough time to grab the ax and split his head open. As he finished killing the first German, the second man returned. Ed axed him to death also, with arterial blood and gore spraying everywhere. He slipped away in the dark, washed in a cold stream, and was able to return to his unit. He was so repulsed by what he had done that he never told any of his comrades what really happened or how he escaped. He told me, "It was intolerable to think about."

During a German counterattack his company was forced to retreat. He would have had to expose himself in the open at close range to retreat with the rest. Instead, he crawled under the bodies of three of his comrades, playing dead as their blood and gore dripped and oozed over him. Several hours later, after his unit drove the Germans off, he "resurrected" from under his comrades' corpses to the surprise of his unit.

In the spring of 1945 his battalion was dug in on the south side of a flooding, northern Italian river. In the foxhole next to him was their battalion commander who had been with them since they came to Italy. He was an officer they all respected for his good sense and courage. The field phone rang. Ed listened to his officer's side of the conversation. It became apparent that they were being ordered to cross the river that night in rubber boats and attack the dug-in German positions on the other side. The officer was adamant that this was pure suicide and that all of them would be killed. They had insufficient men and covering fire for any chance of success. He finally snapped and slammed the phone down. The last Ed saw of him, he was headed to the rear, apparently to confront the man who had given him the order. Ed never saw him again and supposed his commander was court-martialed. He felt this officer's disobedience saved many lives. It was a few days before they had a new commander, and when the attack came there was much better artillery support and covering fire. "You felt like someone had kidnapped your father," was Ed's comment on the loss of this good officer.[1]

In early May 1945 Ed's company entered a small town near the Austrian border. Ed was checking out a two-storey home, searching for Germans.

On the second floor he found the body of a very pregnant young woman who had been tied down nude in a four-poster bed, her hands tied to the head posts, her ankles and knees bound together and tied to one of the bottom posts. The mattress was soaked in blood that had come from her vagina. She and her unborn child had died in labor when her uterus ruptured. She must have suffered horrible agony. He did not know who had done this. It could have been the retreating Nazis. Even more disturbing to Ed, it could have been the anti-Fascist Italians taking heartless revenge on a villager pregnant by a German. "It filled me with a hate and rage I was uncertain I could control." He was all of 19.

Ed bravely served, fought and returned home to help raise a family and make a living as a mailman. By the early 1980s he was still having regular nightmares and intrusive thoughts of the war. One morning his wife found him in the front yard in a foxhole he had dug during the night. His ammo and hunting rifles were placed around him ready to repel an attack. She feared he would have killed anyone who trespassed that night. She insisted he come to the VA hospital for the first time. After I treated him individually for several months, he became a charter member of the first WWII combat vets group I started with a co-therapist.

We had been meeting for about two years and were discussing some of the vets' more distressing experiences in greater depth when Ed said quietly, "Aren't we all murderers?" As I looked around the group, I was sobered and distressed to see many nodding in apparent agreement. I did not know how to respond. But I was able to listen long enough to eventually learn. One of the things I have learned is that Ed's story was not atypical. Nor was his response to what he had done and experienced.

Doug was 16 when he joined the US Army. He and his parents had lied about his age when he joined the service. He explained, "We were poor and it was one less mouth to feed at home." By the time he turned 17, he had been in combat in the "Iron Triangle" in Korea for three weeks. His tough veteran platoon sergeant said, "Do exactly what I say, when I say it, and you might survive and keep some of your buddies alive as well." That included killing any "gooks" that moved, even if they appeared helplessly wounded and seemed to "beg for mercy with their eyes." "Wounded gooks have killed my men. Never let that happen again," was the justification. Doug killed several. One night he killed a Chinese soldier who approached in the dark. He had yelled something in broken English before Doug shot him. "Maybe he was trying to surrender or defect? He didn't have a weapon when I checked him."

As the fighting continued, Doug became an experienced, tough NCO. After several months of intense, grueling combat, he returned to the States. He admitted in group that he was "scared sick" coming home. He could not say why initially. Later he wrote to me and said, "The reason I was afraid getting off the boat coming home in 1952 was I felt like I had left my poor soul in Korea! THAT'S NOT GOOD!" (emphasis by Doug).

Frank was deep in enemy territory, leading a LRRP (long range reconnaissance patrol) in Southeast Asia during the Vietnam War. They unexpectedly encountered a small North Vietnamese unit, and a sharp, brief firefight ensued. Three of his men were mortally wounded and in extreme pain. He gave them what morphine he could. Rescue was impossible. It took another hour for them all to die. At one point each begged Frank to kill him to end his pain, but Frank could not bring himself to do it. Frank remembers each one cursing him for not having the guts to kill them. "At the time it seemed like murder to kill our own. Now I still hear and see their agony and wonder why I didn't have the guts to finish them off. How could I have been so heartless?"

Donald Lopez, who flew fighter planes in combat against the Japanese in China during WWII, describes the actions of an admired officer, who, faced with watching a brave flight engineer suffer terribly as he burned to death in a plane crash, chose an alternative death for him:

The flight surgeon, Dr. Keefe, had arrived, and by crouching behind blankets soaked in muddy water, we were able to get him close enough to the flight engineer to see if he could be freed by amputating a leg. This too was impossible, since he was trapped in the wreckage from the waist down.

By now the fire was completely out of control, and we were forced to break away. The ammunition began to explode, and the machine guns to fire. We backed off still further and were watching helplessly as the fire approached the trapped engineer, who never lost consciousness or, apparently, hope.

Colonel Dunning, Commanding Officer of the Fifth Fighter Group CACW and the ranking officer at Chihkiang, arrived on the scene from the headquarters building. He assessed the situation and asked if there was any way that we could save the engineer. We told him we had tried everything possible, but there was no hope now of saving him.

He walked up as close as possible to the raging fire, drew his .45 pistol, and carefully aimed it at the engineer. At that moment the engineer looked up at Colonel Dunning and said, "Don't shoot me, colonel; I'm going to get out of here." Colonel Dunning holstered his gun, and the engineer, mustering all his strength, raised himself on his arms, as though doing a push-up, and looked down under his body to see what was holding him. While he looked down, Colonel Dunning drew his pistol and shot him in the top of his head, killing him instantly.

... Colonel Dunning never mentioned the incident, but it was obvious that he was strongly affected by it. He was ordered to Kumming to be court-martialed, and every officer and man on base volunteered to testify in his behalf. It was not necessary, as the court-martial was only a formality, done as much to protect him from future prosecution, as to adhere to military regulations.

Colonel Dunning was one of the finest men I have ever known, completely fearless, a brilliant pilot and tactician, and an inspiring leader. He went on to become a brigadier general and would undoubtedly have gone higher had he not died suddenly in 1962, on the operating table from a reaction to the anesthetic. If there is a Valhalla, he is surely there – along with the flight engineer.[2]

Men like Frank and Colonel Dunning are often faced with dreadful options in war. They make the best choices they can at the time but often carry a heavy burden in their hearts for many years after.

Jack was in Special Forces in the US Army Reserves when Desert Storm started. He was young, proud and gung-ho. He wanted a chance to fight for his country and use the skills he had learned. He asked to be activated in the regular Special Forces. The Army was happy to take him, but he was assigned to a supply unit. "These guys just weren't warriors. They were slugs." They were deployed near the front just behind the attacking army units as they moved into Kuwait. Off duty Jack would go on "one man patrols, armed to the teeth." He was stealthily rounding an abandoned bunker when he abruptly confronted an Arab in flowing robes. Jack fired first. The Arab did have a weapon, but nothing on him confirmed he was an enemy. Jack never told anyone what had happened, but he knew he had killed a man the day before the fighting ended. Was he an Iraqi agent? A deserter? A Kuwaiti trying to return home? Had he killed a combatant or murdered an innocent wanderer in no man's land? These questions had been eating at his heart for nine years when he first saw me.

That these men were troubled by symptoms of posttraumatic stress disorder (PTSD) for years if not for decades would not surprise anyone familiar with the field. The American Psychiatric Association's *Diagnostic and Statistical Manual of Mental Disorders*, fourth edition (*DSM-IV*), states that to make the diagnosis a person must have, "... experienced, witnessed, or was confronted with an event or events that involved actual or threatened death ... and the person's response involved intense fear, helplessness, or horror."[3] Certainly this describes part of what happened to these men.

All these combatants (Ed, Doug, Frank and Jack) fit the symptomatic criteria for PTSD.[4] They suffered daily nightmares and intrusive thoughts for years. They struggled with startle reactions to loud noises (fireworks, backfires and so on) and avoided stimuli that reactivated painful memories and emotions (certain movies, war news, various smells). They struggled with emotional numbing and guilt.

This book, however, will not focus on traditional PTSD diagnosis and treatment. Our current PTSD diagnosis is primarily based on the conditioned responses people develop because of their traumatic experiences. These conditioned responses to combat become the most readily recognizable symptoms that continue to trouble vets later. However, my veteran patients have taught me that as troubling as these conditioned responses are (nightmares, intrusive thoughts, startle reactions, and many others), they are not what disturb them most over the course of their lives. What they are most troubled by is the guilt over killing, the traumatic grief they suffer for beloved comrades brutally killed and the fear that they may have let their comrades down at some crucial point. This book will focus primarily on these three issues and what my ordinary combat vets have taught me about their emotional and moral struggles to overcome their guilt and pain. Thus, for the majority of combatants, it is not the basic problems of traditional PTSD that trouble them most (as bad as those are), but the problems of "having bloodstained hands" from various forms of war killing and living with the deep grief engendered by the traumatic loss of men who were "as close as brothers."[5]

Combatants often experience a profound change in how they feel about themselves and the world in general. The nature of their relationships is also deeply altered. Those who knew them before the war always saw significant changes in their loved ones on their return, usually along the lines described by the sister of this WWII Navy vet. She wrote me the following:

After nearly 50 years of suffering silently, Mark is beginning to open up and is talking to us (his family) about some of his experiences – at least enough that we are starting to understand the changes in attitude towards family and the uncharacteristic silence about what was bothering him that was so hard for us to comprehend all these years. Mark was, by nature, anything but a quiet youngster. He was the life of the party – involved in every activity available in our area: high school all state quarterback, Golden Glove champion of the western states, cowboy, all-around good brother: he always saved his sisters a dance, gave us money, drove us places. He was protective of us. Content with his life ... The combat years were very different. His letters began to focus on just letting us know he was alive – and trying to tell us where he was ... When he finally returned home after the war, Mark was not the same brother. He was quiet, restless and very nervous. He never talked about the war experiences, didn't stay around home very much. He acted like he wanted to be alone; and he seemed to feel that nobody gave a damn about what he had been through (Of course, we had no idea what that was because he wouldn't talk about it.).

In this letter, Mark's sister eloquently describes the experience of nearly every family that has had a combatant return from war.

Combatants often change spiritually as well. Ed's wife explained how her husband had changed:

We were regular churchgoers before the war. He was a good Christian. He never could understand after the war how God could forgive him for all he had seen and done. It changed our life in that respect. He felt like a hypocrite going to church. We tried to go together for a while, but he was just too uncomfortable.

Although John Hersey is best known as a Pulitzer Prize winning novelist, he also served as a war correspondent in WWII. Like Ernie Pyle, he spent his time close to the front writing about the men who day to day were killing and dying. In the preface to a collection of his war reports published in 1945 he notes, "... these are stories of what common men, not necessarily leaders or heroes, feel as they wage war – and their feelings are inevitably reduced, in the end, to what men cannot help feeling about their worst crime, which is murder."[6]

To my surprise I have found, as John Hersey suggests, that even fifty years later many common soldiers who fought and killed in war struggle with a deep inner burden that they may in some fashion be guilty of murder. Before I started working with combat vets, I imagined that the fear of being killed was the hardest thing to face in war. Fear of death is difficult to face and conquer, but for most men the loathing of killing is even harder to overcome. After the war some men are troubled by having not done their duty due to fear, but far more are troubled by having killed. How, then, did they initially get to the point where they could kill and how were they able to continue doing it?

Notes

1 In a similar episode Brendan Phibbs describes watching his West Point colonel refuse a direct command in order to save his men from certain death as they faced the Germans in Europe in WWII. (*The Other Side of Time*, pp. 138–40, 148. For a second episode of the same see p. 151.)
2 Lopez, Donald, *Into the Teeth of the Tiger*. pp. 220–3.
3 *Diagnostic and Statistical Manual of Mental Disorders Fourth Edition*, pp. 427–8. Published by the American Psychiatric Association, Washington, DC, 1994.
4 Ibid pp. 427–9.
5 Lopez, op. cit. pp. 54, 229.
6 Hersey, John, *Of Men and War*, Introduction.

Chapter 2

How Propaganda and Love Make War Possible

Aggression, Propaganda and War

In the two pieces of mixed media art shown below, Myke Knutson, a Vietnam combat veteran, expresses some of his inner feelings about the nightmare of war as he experienced it. In the first, a Vietcong AK-47 is spattered with the blood it is meant to spill – forcing us to acknowledge the weapon's true purpose. For the artist this AK-47 image is a metaphor of all weapons of war. [Figure 2.1]

The second painting is a self-portrait. The artist shows both his enemies and himself as skeletal "grim reapers," harvesting death with the tools of battle. Part of the harvest is the child's head contained in his satchel. The medal on his chest and the phrase "birth control" mock those who glorify war. [Figure 2.2]

The artist and those noted in Chapter 1 all served their country honorably and continued to work and cope after the war, yet aspects of their experiences still haunt them. They are often troubled most by the killing they have done. Put yourself in their boots. There are so many ways to kill in war. You cannot escape it. If you are in a combat unit and you do not kill the enemy, then the enemy kills you. Or, even worse, he kills others you love (yes, love) in your unit, and you then are responsible for their deaths. If your unit (submarine, plane, platoon) kills, and you support the actions of the unit, then you know you participated in the killing as well, even if you didn't fire the torpedoes, drop the bombs, or pull the trigger.

It is not easy to get men to kill. Studies from WWII suggest that no more than 15–20 per cent of men would kill.[1] The job of a good combat officer or NCO was to find out who in the unit would kill and put those men on the heavy weapons. My work with vets has confirmed this. But any decent, thinking man knows that when he passes ammunition to the man pulling the trigger, he is participating in the killing also.

Arly was in his 60s when he first came to see me. He had been referred for treatment of "anxiety." By this point I had treated hundreds of combat

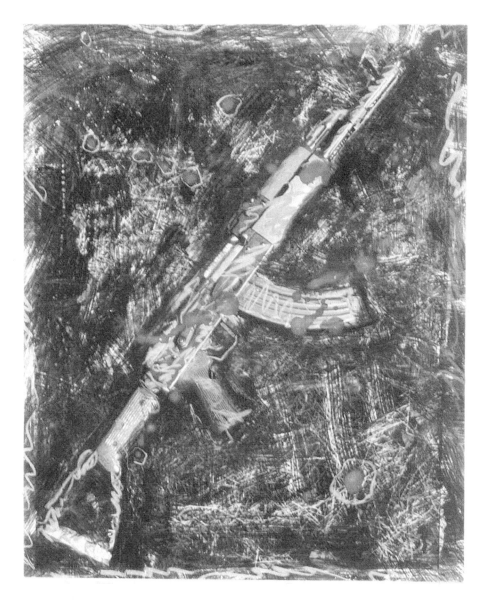

Figure 2.1   Vietcong AK-47

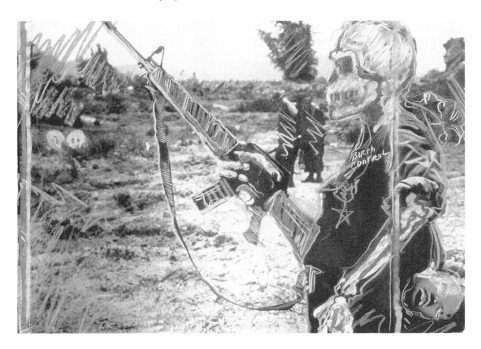

Figure 2.2   Self-portrait of a combatant

vets for many years and could often sense when they were carrying a burden they needed to share. Arly initially stated that he just wanted medication and did not want to talk about the war. Over the next several sessions we danced around what troubled him most. Finally I said, "Arly, did you ever kill anyone?" A tortured "NO!" exploded from his lips. He had never discussed the killing before. However, as our sessions continued, he revealed, "I killed everyone my squad killed. If I hadn't been there, my squad would all be dead. A few would never fire more than into the air. The rest would point in the general direction of the enemy and close their eyes and pull the trigger. They would risk their lives for each other, but they would not kill. I killed a lot of Germans up close to keep us alive." After three months in combat Arly was seriously wounded and evacuated to England, never to return to the war. "I felt guilty, wondering how my squad kept alive after I was gone."

Despite the picture often painted in the media, it is very hard to get men to kill each other; and kill each other they must or war is not possible. And as long as at least one group is willing to kill to attain power, all others must respond in kind or be the victims of the ruthless. I have learned from my veteran patients that both propaganda and love are necessary to begin and continue the killing that makes war possible. How do propaganda and love work to make war happen?

In his powerful treatise, *On Aggression*, Nobel Prize winning biologist Conrad Lorenz discusses the types of aggression found in the animal kingdom. He points out that intra-species aggression is usually modulated and ritualized in such a way that competing males rarely hurt each other. For example, bull elk are awesome creatures. With their powerful hooves, antlers, and great strength they can defend themselves against anything in the forest, even a grizzly bear. Yet when they vie for dominance, they rarely harm each other, but carefully lock horns and then begin pushing each other around. The strongest prevails in this careful test of power, and the weaker leaves the scene. If they were ruthlessly aggressive, they would probably both be mortally wounded. A similar scenario plays out in most other intra-species struggles over sex and territory.

The same is true for the social creature called man. Lorenz argues that the most we would usually do is get involved in fisticuffs, if bluffing and strutting failed.[2] Human aggression is naturally muted by our "parliament" of social instincts.[3] Our greatest evolutionary strength is our ability to plan, share and work together. Too much intra-species aggression works against our survival.

Unfortunately we have added weapons that kill at a distance and at great speed, requiring no more effort than pushing a button or pulling a trigger. We don't necessarily even have to look into the faces and eyes of our enemy. Yet the consequences of pushing a button or pulling a trigger can overwhelm us with remorse and guilt when we see the cost in others' flesh.

It is natural for us to kill other species for food. Having grown up hunting and fishing, I do not feel aggressive when I shoot and eat a deer or catch and eat a trout. In the culture of my youth, hunting and fishing were enjoyable ways to supplement our usual diet. But as Lorenz notes, there are two forms of interspecies aggression – "mobbing" and the "critical reaction" – that can play into the killing of war.[4] Both occur when a weaker species defends itself against its natural predators.

Mobbing is a behavior seen when a weaker species very aggressively tries to defend itself from a predator. I see it every spring outside my window at work. We have a pair of great horned owls that return to nest each year in a large elm tree on the Boise VAMC grounds. These powerful predators are at the peak of the avian food chain in our area. Yet the local ravens gather in self-defense and try to drive them away with constant cawing, careful swooping and aggressive harassment – probably in an instinctive attempt to get them to nest elsewhere. I was watching one day, as one of the "mob" got too close to the perched owl. A powerful claw darted out and seized the raven; a powerful beak decapitated it and dropped it to the ground. The aggressive mob was not deterred but kept a more respectful distance. Humans also can feel threatened by a predator and experience the aggressive feelings spawned by this fear. These feelings can lead to aggressive group action against the predator.

The second form of aggression acted out in war is the "critical reaction" or "cornered rat syndrome." It could also be called the "cornered cat syndrome." It is displayed when a predator traps a small, spunky animal. In a desperate struggle to survive, unable to flee, it launches itself at the face of its larger attacker, snarling and spitting to try to bluff and fight its way to freedom. This aggressive and violent defensive reaction is also activated when the animals' brood, litter or family is threatened and cannot successfully flee from the predator.[5] The parent often appears completely willing to sacrifice itself to protect its young.

Mobbing and the critical reaction are types of defensive aggression spawned by fear. The greater the fear the prey has of the perceived predator or attacker, the more aggressive the response. It is one of the ironies of war that both sides usually see their war as an act of self-defense, even if they are the side that makes the first lethal assault. Most humans will only fight in self-defense. The key to activating a willingness to aggressively defend ourselves to the point of bloodshed is to convince us that we have no other real alternative. It is fight or die. Persuasive propaganda can help push us to that conclusion.

One of the core efforts of propaganda is to convince us that the enemy is not really a human who can be safely reasoned with and accommodated, but is a merciless monster of another species. We must kill this predator or be killed. We are defending ourselves, families, tribe, nation or race against this inhuman or subhuman other. There is no crime in killing a savage or subhuman beast trying to kill us. This attitude, plus the rapid and long distance killing made possible through modern weapons, makes it easier to begin the process of war.

The enemy is inhuman and monstrous. He is the Nazi, the Hun, the Gook, the Commie, the greedy Capitalist, the Terrorist, or the Infidel. He is choking off our economic and political life, threatening our physical existence and subverting our spiritual values. The enemy tortures, pillages, rapes and murders. There might be some elements of truth in the stereotype, but in the end a whole people is usually demonized. As can be seen by close inspection of the WWII propaganda cited and in some cases illustrated below, all sides portray "the other" as less than human while portraying themselves as noble and good. The message is always the same. We are cornered and must fight to remain free from this demonic group that is trying to enslave or destroy us. It is kill or be killed, or worse – become enslaved and let our women be raped and tortured.

Each side in the conflict portrays themselves as noble, strong and good. A racist national philosophy or belief system, such as the Nazi doctrine of Aryan superiority or the Japanese belief in their own divine descent and purity, makes it even easier to justify attacking and killing lesser mortals. When they go to war, they portray themselves as only doing what they have to do to defend themselves and others from the depraved and monstrous enemy. This is illustrated by juxtaposing the Nazi SS recruitment poster with the Nazi view of England led by Churchill as a greedy octopus.[6] [Figures 2.3 and 2.4] It is seen again in the Nazi dogma that leads to the Holocaust – simply purifying Germany by cleaning out an infestation of Jewish "bats."[7] [Figure 2.5] Two Italian Fascist recruitment posters illustrate the same point. They are recruiting the best kind of humans to fight the Neanderthal-like Americans who are going to rape and pillage Italy if given the chance.[8] The Japanese, of course, are no less noble in sending their sons to fight for the freedom of Asia and save Juan of the Philippines from the "sharks of American imperialism and racial prejudice."[9]

The main thrust of the propaganda, though, is that the enemy, even if human, is too cold, heartless, criminal or angry to be negotiated with. Fighting back is our only real option. This is clearly seen in American posters depicting Tojo as a cannibalistic beast and a more realistic, but merciless, Japanese soldier preparing to fire his rifle.[10] [Figure 2.6] It is also seen in American posters about the Nazis. One shows the unfeeling face of a sadistic German officer and another portrays a German victory as bringing slavery and death for America, just as it did for Czechoslovakia.[11] [Figure 2.7]

The bottom line is "Kill the Fascist beast" before he rapes and kills the women of Russia; stop the two headed "monster" of Tojo and Hitler before they destroy America; and cut off the claw-like hands of Germany and Japan before they grasp the beautiful women and children of Canada.[12] [Figures 2.8, 2.9 and 2.10] There is no rational alternative but to fight and kill the enemy.

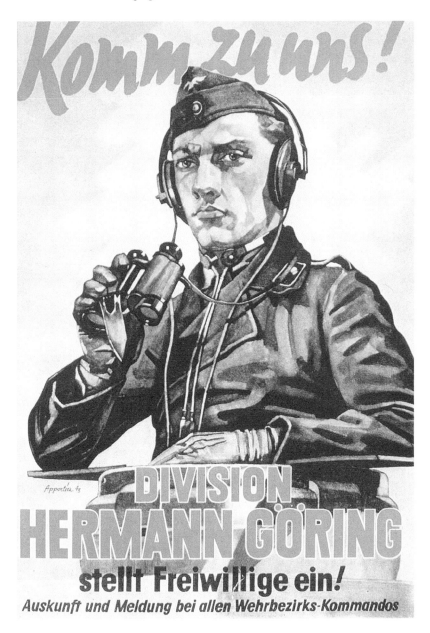

Figure 2.3   Nazi SS recruitment poster

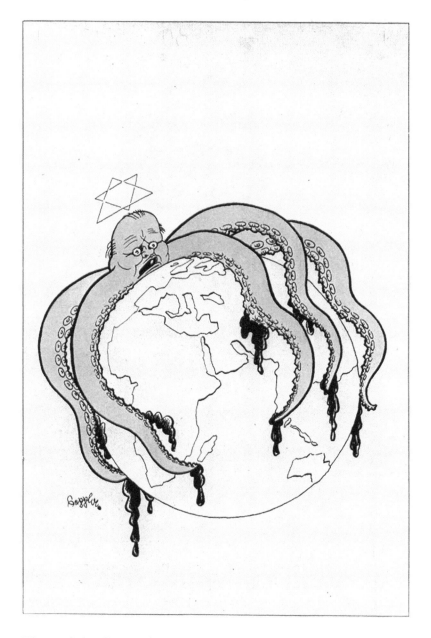

Figure 2.4   Churchill as a greedy Jewish octopus

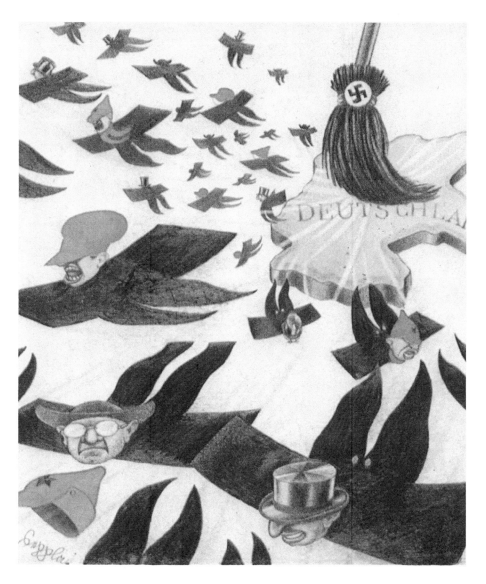

Figure 2.5   Purging Germany of Jewish bats

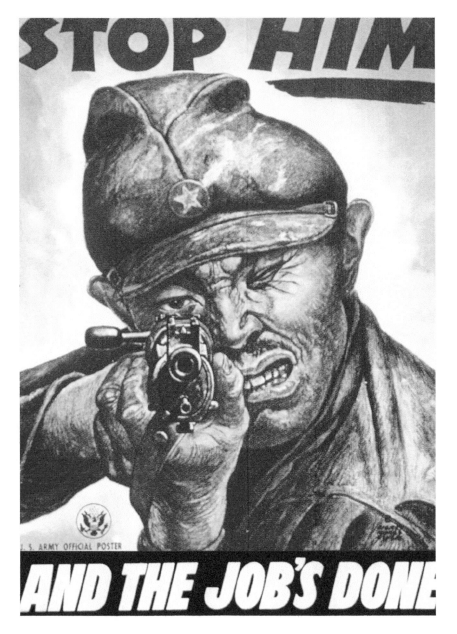

Figure 2.6   Merciless Japanese soldier

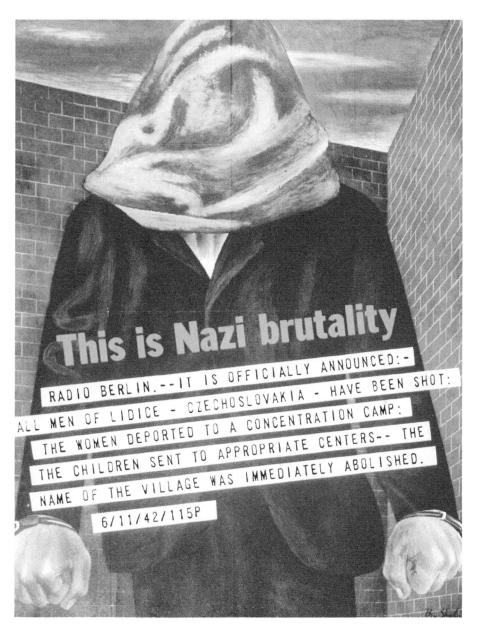

Figure 2.7 Results of a Nazi victory

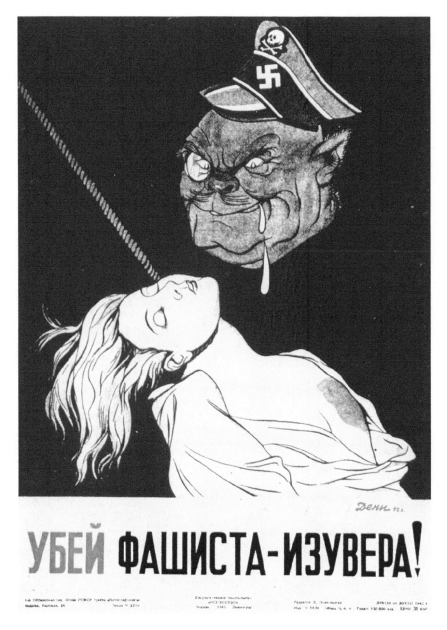

Figure 2.8   Kill the Fascist beast

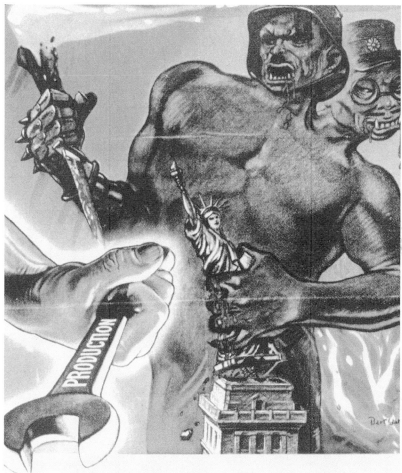

Figure 2.9   Stop this monster

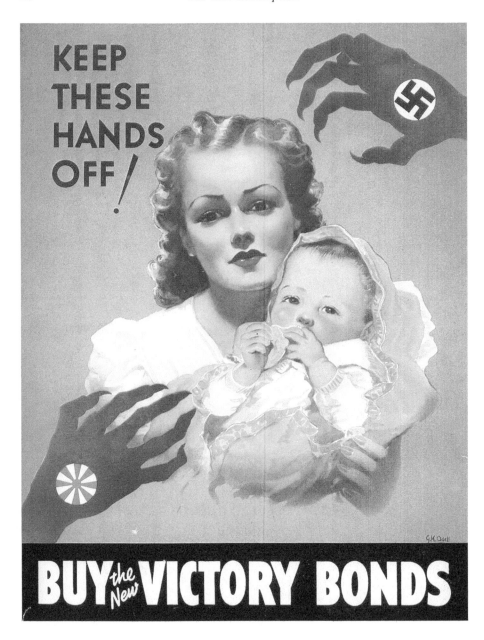

Figure 2.10   Save the women and children of Canada

Late one evening in 1995 I was watching a TV special aired as part of the celebration of the 50th anniversary of the end of World War II. A prominent history professor stated that the USA only dropped the atom bomb on Japan because we were racist; we would have never used it on the Germans in Europe. He seemed unwilling to consider the possibility that A-bombs may have saved more lives than they destroyed by bringing the war to a swifter conclusion;[13] and he obviously had never dug into the minds of the WWII generation. For that generation the Nazis were just as horrible monsters as were the "Japs." The Nazis enslaved Europe and perpetrated the Holocaust. The British Royal Air Force fire-bombed German cities almost every night for two years, while the US Army Air Force bombed them in the daylight. The firebombing of Dresden in the spring of 1945 killed more civilians than the second A-bomb on Nagasaki. If it had been ready in time, we would have used the atom bomb to bring the war to a swifter conclusion in Europe. Luckily for some, Germany surrendered before the A-bomb was ready. Unfortunately for those involved on both sides in Normandy, the Bulge and the conventional bombing of Germany, and for those in the Nazi death camps during the last months of the war in Europe, the A-bomb was not ready in time to shorten the war and spare the hundreds of thousands killed in conventional ways on both sides in those last months of WWII in Europe.

The professor was missing the larger point. War, by nature, is racist. We have to be fighting dangerous "animals," not other feeling, caring humans. When we have been demonized, we often have no choice but to mount our own propaganda campaign and get the "cornered rat" hormones and adrenalin flowing to defend ourselves. Most people cannot think of the enemy as decent humans and still kill them. As one of my vets, Larry – who ambushed and killed the enemy up close many times – expressed it, "I had to pretend I was killing a cobra – coiled to strike. If I didn't, it was almost impossible to take that first shot. Once the shooting starts, your instincts to protect your men and stay alive take over and help you finish the killing."

Sometimes the propaganda and the distance from the dead and dying protect the combatants from the immediate emotional impact of killing other humans. During Desert Storm I stayed up late watching C-SPAN broadcast an interview with two handsome young American flyers. They had helped to rout the Iraqi Republican Guard from their occupation of Kuwait. They flew A-10 Warthogs and had spent the day destroying more than 30 Iraqi tanks. The reporters crowded around asking the kind of bland, inane questions sports writers usually ask athletes. Then a grizzled, older reporter who looked like a Vietnam combat vet to my clinical eyes said, "What do you think about the Iraqis you killed today?" It was quiet for a moment as the two pilots looked at each other, and then the senior in rank replied, "I don't think we killed any today. As we circled over the battlefield, you could see them bailing out of those tanks and running before we ever fired."

Unfortunately for these two men, that belief would not be sustainable. Within a few days the media was showing footage of the burning tanks and charred bodies that clogged the roads from Kuwait City to Iraq. The enemy body count would be staggering (possibly as many as 100 000) and the charred, dismembered bodies would be clearly recognizable as human, as would be the defeated faces of the thousands of prisoners of war, very few of whom did anything more than "defend their country."

A pilot who helped destroy the Japanese aircraft carriers and other ships at the Battle of Midway in WWII describes a turning point in his feelings about what he was doing. He was elated as he watched his bombs help destroy those ships that had launched the attack on Pearl Harbor. Later he flew low over the fantail of a cruiser as it was sinking. As the "mass of people" looked up at him, he felt "sudden sympathy for their helplessness." For him a "hated enemy" had "become a pitied human being."[14]

One of my WWII vets, a local farmer, describes, "the biggest mistake I ever made" this way:

> I was a machine gunner. We had been fighting to retake Guam for several days and the battle in our area was nearing its conclusion. About one hundred yards away eleven Japanese jumped up and charged our position in broad daylight. I mowed them down like hay – surprised they made it so easy as they usually were wily and skilled soldiers. When it was clear nothing else was happening, I crept out with a couple of buddies to field strip them and get some souvenirs. First we found they had no ammo. All their rifles were empty. They had used us to commit suicide rather than surrender. Then I made the biggest mistake I ever made in the war. I pulled the wallet out of one man's pocket and opened it. Inside was a picture of a beautiful young woman and little girl, about the same age as my wife and daughter. That image has haunted me to this day.

A Marine rifleman was working as a scout sifting through papers from dead Japanese soldiers on a rainy day toward the end of the campaign on Okinawa. He had fought through Peleliu and Okinawa in the South Pacific, and up to that point had only hate for the Japanese. He describes how that changed as he and his buddy searched a dead officer, hoping to find something useful for their intelligence unit:

I handed Tony a soggy wallet stuffed with papers. We spread a poncho on the ground and began to sort through the papers – the biggest lump of them were pictures and letters. There was a picture of a dignified old Japanese gentleman.

"Father," Tony said.

There was a picture of a broad-faced lady still with jet-black hair. "Mother," Tony said.

There was a younger woman in full kimono and obi. "Wife or sweetheart," Tony said.

There was a picture of a chubby, black-eyed boy. "Kid," Tony said. "Then it must have been wife – the young one, I mean. Handsome kid, isn't he?"

At that moment, for the first time in the war, I felt pity for the enemy. On Peleliu we had seen few enemy dead. They had been dragged into caves by their mates or sealed in bunkers by our demolitionists. On Okinawa I had seen hundreds of dead, but I felt nothing toward them until we searched the Japanese in the gully and found the pictures of his wife and child. Then I realized that we were killing other humans who fathered children and had parents who loved them, just as we had ... From that day in the rain I never again hated the Japanese. I just wished that the war would end so we could stop killing each other.[15]

Sooner or later the soldier recognizes that the other guy he is trying to kill is just that, another guy like him. Then he can no longer kill with impunity, and that particular burden of war begins to mount. We will explore this more throughout the book, but we now turn to another powerful force that makes war possible – love.

Love and War

My introduction to the role love plays in war occurred well before I ever went to medical school. While living in France during my college years, I visited a large WWII American cemetery in eastern France, searching for the grave of my cousin who had been killed in the Battle of the Bulge. I didn't find his grave that day, but I did find the citations of three Medal of Honor recipients who were buried there. More than 30 years later I remember neither their names nor the name of the cemetery, but I remember their stories.

The first soldier was decorated for an action in Italy and later killed in combat in France. A lieutenant with a Ranger unit, he was leading a two-jeep reconnaissance patrol. They rounded a curve in the road and came face to face with two German tanks. He leapt off the first jeep with his Tommy gun and grenades and ran directly at the tanks, ordering his men to flee.

Fortunately for him, he caught the tank crews unprepared and was able to destroy both tanks by throwing grenades down their hatches before they could button up, start their engines, and become battle ready. He obviously was willing to sacrifice his life to buy a little time for his men to get clear. He was also willing to kill to save them.

The second Medal of Honor winner was a medic whose company had walked into a minefield in the fog. He spent several hours crawling in and out of the minefield rescuing his wounded men. He eventually was wounded by a mine but continued his rescue efforts until he died of his wounds. His life apparently did not mean as much to him as saving the lives of the men he loved.

The third man was a platoon leader in Patton's 3rd US Army as they drove across France. His men, pinned down by a German machine gun, could neither safely advance nor retreat without fully exposing themselves to withering fire. As it was, they were slowly being killed. Finally he rushed the machine gun nest and, catching them reloading, killed the three-man crew. This scenario repeated itself several more times in the next few weeks. The platoon ended up in Metz. A few hundred German SS troopers were surrounded in the town hall and wouldn't surrender. American tanks were drawn up on all sides to flatten the building and kill the Germans. This lieutenant begged his commanding officer to let him try to negotiate with these "Nazi fanatics." Risking his life again, but this time for the enemy, he went in under a white flag and eventually persuaded them to surrender.

To me all these men's actions seemed motivated by love. "Was that typical for war?" I wondered at the time. It seemed so incongruous with what I thought war was about. I had much to learn.

JR walked into my office crying. His primary care physician referred him to me because "he can't stop crying and doesn't know why." After an hour talking to him, I didn't know why either. He was neither hallucinating nor delusional. He was not suicidal or classically depressed. He was not panic stricken. He agreed to come and see me again in two days.

He was still softly crying when I saw him next. "I get up and within a few minutes I am crying again, and it continues until I go to sleep." This had been going on for three months. I began taking a detailed military history. In the next hour we hit pay dirt. JR had formally retired from his civilian career several months previously. A few months later he had started crying, 41 years to the day – the exact anniversary – of his last bombing mission over Germany.

I was 32 years old. Most of the boys on the B-17 were teenagers. I was older than the pilots, and as a senior sergeant I was like a father to them. They came to me with all their troubles and worries. That last mission was a nightmare. I have always tried to forget it but never really could. There were eleven of us on the plane. Our plane was riddled by machine gun fire from fighters and shrapnel from flak. I was wounded in the foot, but put a tourniquet on it and just kept going. Two engines were shot out. All of us but one were wounded. As we tried to make it back to England, I crawled around the plane trying to patch them up and keep them alive. Some died crying in my arms. It broke my heart.

JR was evacuated from the field hospital in England to a hospital in Plattsburg, New York. The parents of five of his "dead boys" were within a day's travel. When he had recovered sufficiently, he went to see them all. "I shouldn't have done it. To see their grief, and for me to be alive and their sons dead, was just too much. I've tried to put it out of my mind ever since." The tears he was shedding when he came to me were from simple, deep grief – sadness over the brutal, intimate deaths of men he loved like his own sons. Deaths and losses for which he had never finished grieving. Two weeks later when I started my first WWII PTSD group, he, like Ed, was a charter member. I always kidded him that he finally got me off the dime and doing the job I needed to do. JR, Ed, and the men in that first group continued my education on the role of love in war.

A few years later I was giving a lecture on PTSD to our local medical society. After the lecture an older physician came up to me and said he had a book he thought I would find useful. Some days later he brought me an aged, bound government manual entitled *Psychiatric Experiences of the Eighth Air Force, First Year of Combat (July 4, 1942–July 4, 1943)*. Stamped all over it were the words "RESTRICTED" and "NOT TO BE REPUBLISHED" in bold type. He actually took it out from under the trench coat he was wearing that rainy day, saying, "You can't copy this. I took it from the military when I left at the end of WWII and I don't want anyone to know!" Eventually he did let me copy it, and now we have both revealed to the world what once was a "RESTRICTED" document, but all for a greater good!

I have treated many survivors of the air war over Germany – from the 8th, 15th, 12th, and 9th US Air Forces – and the book has been invaluable in helping me understand their experiences and better care for them. The three psychiatrists who authored it, Major Donald W. Hastings, Captain David G. Wright, and Captain Bernard C. Glueck, provide clinical cases, data and experiences that would help any clinician dealing with war trauma.

One of them even went on a bombing mission "just to better understand what the men were going through" and describes it in detail.[16] Before we look at some of their cases, to better understand what these combatants went through and how love made their successful service possible, it is important to understand some of the basic facts about the 8th and 15th US Air Forces during WWII.

The 8th and 15th US Air Forces conducted daylight bombing raids over Germany, France and other parts of German-occupied Europe. These were to be precision raids – hitting important industrial and military targets. The top secret Norden bombsight allowed the American B-17 and B-24 bombers to accurately bomb targets from 20,000 plus feet. The raids deep into Europe in 1942–43 were conducted without fighter escort. It was not until early 1944, when the P-51 Mustang fighter was deployed and equipped with auxiliary external fuel tanks, that the Allied air forces had a fighter with sufficient range to accompany the bombers to most targets in Germany, Austria and Romania. The military dogma was that the B-17s and B-24s, if they stayed in proper formation, would have sufficient combined firepower from their .50 caliber top, tail, ball turret and waist guns to fight off the German fighter attacks. Although they shot down many German fighters, this dogma proved incorrect. Two thirds of the American bomber crews that first year (July 1942–July 1943) were wounded, captured or killed. Fighter attacks killed most, but flak, "so thick you could walk on it," as some of my vets have described it, took its share. During the entire war the American bomber crews and their fighter escorts in Europe suffered 49,000 men killed, and another 30,000 became prisoners of war (POWs).[17] The nearly 80,000 dead and captured for the US Army Air Force in Europe in WWII totals 20,000 more than the Americans killed and captured in the entire Vietnam War.

On a standard mission the men arose before dawn, ate breakfast, and then reported to the briefing room, which was a large hall with a big blackboard covered by a curtain. The group commander or the intelligence officer would then come out and open the curtain, exposing the blackboard where the mission was outlined. My vets tell me that airmen would start vomiting in nauseous anticipation when they saw where they were expected to fly that day. They were required to fly 25 missions (eventually this was raised to 35) as a tour of duty. Losses were often 10 per cent of the planes per mission, with a much higher percentage damaged. The German air defences were probably the most effective faced by any group of flyers.[18] The American airmen realized after a few missions that their chances of surviving 25 missions were very low. Nevertheless 98–99 per cent of the men kept getting in the planes and flying the missions. Why? My vets have always answered, "You would never let down the men you loved and respected and who loved and respected you."

What follows are three typical cases taken verbatim from this "TOP SECRET" manual. The cases are italicized but my own explanatory comments are not.

Case one. 2nd Lieutenant, Bombardier, B-17, Age 26
Chief Complaint: "Jittery and Depressed"
Present Illness: The officer has been on 19 operational missions from European Theatre of Operations US Army. On the second raid his plane was badly damaged. He states that the plastics nose [This is where the bombardier sits with the bombsight.] *was riddled in a sieve-like fashion by an aerial bomb which filled the nose with smoke and cut him on the hands. The hydraulics on the plane were also shot out. On getting back to base he felt shaky and nervous and that night couldn't sleep for thinking about what he had been through. On this raid he saw his first Fortress* [B-17s were known as Flying Fortresses.] *go down. The next raid was Emden where they encountered heavy flak, had several holes shot in the wings, and he saw a B-17 receive a direct hit, disintegrate, and go down in pieces without any parachutes opening up. On the return he was again shaky, nervous and couldn't sleep. Two days later he went on another raid to Germany, and developed oxygen trouble which scared him* [They all needed oxygen masks because of the high altitude of their missions.]. *It was a rough raid, his plane was damaged to the point of being unserviceable for future raids. Several days later on a raid to France he saw the plane in which his Squadron Commander was pilot, receive severe fighter attack, do an uncontrolled loop and collide with two other B-17's and spin down. His own plane received some flak hits. On return to base he felt nervous and shaky but says he avoided going to the doctor because he didn't want to give up. On the next raid to Bremen, heavy flak was encountered and many fighters met them on the way home, and he saw their wing plane spin in and crash into the sea. His best friend was aboard. The Kiel raid was his worst. His gun was frozen* [It was often so cold that any moisture at all could freeze and jam the moving parts of the machine guns.] *and he sat helplessly watching repeated fighter attacks and heavy flak. The plane in which there was a General was on his wing and he saw it crippled and spin down through the clouds over the target. No one got out that he saw. In rather quick succession on his plane the tail gunner passed out from anoxia, all but 2 guns froze, the No.2 engine was hit and caught fire and the plane on the other wing was hit, went out of control and side-slipped directly underneath them so close that the pilot of his plane had to pull up sharply to avoid a crash. This plane then crashed into the B-17 on their opposite side; they had to do evasive action to miss the pieces of B-17's that were flying in the air. He saw the ball turret* [The ball turret was an exposed,

rotating plastic bubble on the bottom of the plane with twin .50 cal. machine guns and a gunner strapped in a harness. If the hydraulics were knocked out from shrapnel, a frequent occurrence, the gunner could not get out on his own. He had to be cranked out by another crewman. Only a small man with a big hero's heart could stand it.] *knocked off and go down "like an apple" with the gunner still inside. He saw another man jump with a burning parachute and fall "like a hunk of lead." Shortly after another neighboring ship did a loop and spun in. He saw another lose its wings and the fuselage go down end over end, no parachutes being seen. He saw another snap-roll and one wing came off. His own plane was badly damaged and had to be salvaged after this raid. On coming in to land after this raid, the plane ground looped in landing. This raid was a disastrous one for his Group. Ten out of nineteen planes failed to return, the remainder were well shot up, and several including his own were wrecked on landing, the General was missing, and everyone was stunned by what had happened. The patient felt pent-up and restless during the interrogation* [Post-mission, intelligence officers always interviewed all the participants to produce a coherent picture of what happened on the mission for later analysis.], *and after it began crying and weeping. That night in the barracks he broke down again while the clothes of his missing room-mates were being packed up. He tried drinking to relieve his anxiety but it didn't help much. That night he had his first battle dreams, couldn't sleep because of the vivid nightmares of crashing and falling and one time woke up sweating profusely and was told he had been yelling and screaming in his sleep. This raid marked the onset of a severe nervous state and by now throughout the day and night he was tense, tired, depressed, things seemed unreal, and he had difficulty concentrating. A few days later while going to a mission (abortive) he broke down and cried in the truck taking him to the plane and vomited up his breakfast. He states that he did not report his trouble because he felt that he should have enough guts to continue. He was upset by replacement crews that came in after the Kiel raid and said it depressed him to see all the new officers in his friends' beds. On the next raid, he went to Bremen and they couldn't find the target. Eleven ships got separated from the main mass, his among them, and they got down to 12,000 feet over the German coast to bomb a convoy, but he got rattled, forgot to throw on the switch, with the result that all of his bombs hung up* [meaning they didn't drop out of the bomb bay properly]. *This raid, and his bombing failure in it, made him worse. His concentration was gone, he became vague, had dizzy spells and headaches, was jittery, became very irritable, depressed. "I couldn't get a hold of myself." On his last raid to France he "went to pieces," couldn't concentrate and felt muddled trying to adjust his bomb sight. Acting as lead bombardier* [When the lead bombardier dropped his bombs everyone else was to drop theirs as well.] *he "just let the bombs go" and missed the target by 6 miles. He saw some blow up farmhouses which distressed him. Attacked by fighters, he shot his gun without aiming. His symptoms got worse and he had headaches and dizzy spells. On his return to the field he felt he was incapable of acting as bombardier. He told his pilot who tried to reassure him by taking him on practice bombing runs. This did not help any. He made so many foolish mistakes and felt so distressed inside himself that he consulted his Squadron Flight Surgeon who sent him to the Central Medical Board.*

Psychiatric Examination: The patient was obviously tense and anxious, had trouble in talking without his voice wavering, seemed vague, abstract, and preoccupied. His hands trembled to the point where he had difficulty in lighting a cigarette with ease. His shirt was wet under the armpits and he fidgeted in the chair. He stated, almost apologetically, that he is restless, feels distressed and depressed and that he is afraid to go to sleep because of nightmares of combat. He felt that he is "washed up" as far as flying is concerned and will have to do ground duty only. He did not want to go back to his station because there were too many reminders that distressed him.[19]

This flyer's experience is very typical in many respects. Notice how long he held on before he actually became dysfunctional as a combatant. It took the death of the majority of the men in his group, including his closest friend and bunkmates, plus his growing feeling that his symptoms were threatening the success of their efforts, before he sought a way out. He tried drinking. He was not sleeping. The missions were coming in rapid succession and he was exhausted. He finally was formally diagnosed with "operational fatigue" and grounded. He was treated and returned to duty, but not to combat.

Case two: T/Sgt., Tail Gunner, B-17, Age 26
Chief Complaint: "Fear of Flying"
Present Illness: The patient is a tail gunner on a B-17. On October 2, 1942 they were flying on a practice mission at 26,000 feet and the waist gunner passed out because of anoxia. The pilot put the ship into a vertical dive [This was done to get the anoxic gunner rapidly to a lower altitude and hopefully save his life.] and tried to pull out at approximately 20,000 feet. The cables snapped, the right wing and engines pulled off, and the plane caught on fire. The bomb bay doors flew off and apparently one of them hurtled backwards and sliced off the tail section at the region of the tail gunner's escape hatch. The patient in the tail section went hurtling down end over end. The patient tried to smash his way out through the glass and failed and then kicked his way through the skin of the ship and wiggled through but his shoulders became wedged. He must have been blown clear at about 1000 feet and had time to get his parachute open before hitting the ground. He was unharmed. The only other survivor, a gunner, parachuted down nearby but was injured. The plane had crashed about 100 yards from where the patient landed in the midst of a

British anti-aircraft battery and was burning. The patient and several British soldiers ran over to the burning fuselage and tried to pull one of the men out through the waist window but it was apparent that he was crushed and dead. Because of the fire they backed away and shortly after the plane exploded and burning gasoline created a large fire. The patient then went back and called the Commanding Officer to report the accident. The accident occurred at dusk and it was about 1900 hours before he could get the telephone call through. He went to bed at a nearby British station and almost all night lay sweating, shaking, tense and restless. The following morning he felt "jittery" and "ill at ease," and went out to the wreck with the Commanding Officer and the medical officer. There he saw the charred bodies of the other 8 men in the plane. For the following 2 days he couldn't eat. Since the accident he has felt tense, anxious and restless. He sleeps poorly and has frequently recurring dreams of plane crashes. He has difficulty in getting thoughts of crashes off his mind and little things remind him of it. He develops anxiety on getting into the forward section of a B-17 because it reminds him of the terrible experience his fellow crew members must have gone through before the crash killed them. Whistling and whining noises startle him because they remind him of the wind whistling through the jagged tail section as it fell from the wreck. Small enclosed spaces also produce a certain amount of anxiety. The nights when he is alone are his worst time. He feels better in the day when he can talk to other people and have their company. He has developed severe anxiety attacks on riding in planes since the accident and says he sits listening to the creaking of the plane waiting for the tail section to break off again. In spite of these symptoms he has flown 5 operational missions since the accident. In two of these he went through further terrifying experiences in seeing his plane badly hit by flak and on one of these occasions it had to come home on 2 motors with a badly torn wing and lacerated fuselage [My vets love to argue about which plane was better, B-17 or B-24, but all agree that the B-17 could take tremendous damage and still get home.]. *On this mission while acting as waist gunner flak blew pieces of canvas over his head and into his mouth and wrapped some control cables around his neck. This occurred over the target and he states he was so frightened that he almost bailed out without orders. He states that he did not report these symptoms to the medical officer but went on forcing himself to fly, when several days ago he was instructed to report to the Central Medical Board. He stated that he does not wish to be regarded as "yellow" or a "quitter" but now that the thing has come to a head, he states that he never wants to get into an airplane again. It might be added that on one of the missions a F.W.190* [a German fighter plane] *appeared 50 feet behind his tail turret and the patient saw his tracer bullets enter where the oxygen bottles are located. There was a flash of flame and the German spun down out of control. This increased the patient's anxiety because he felt in a way that he had been responsible for causing another man to go through an experience like he had gone through ... Since the accident he has received a letter from his wife stating she is pregnant. The patient states that his wife and mother are unaware of the fact that he has done any operational flying, and that he has never told them he is a regular member of a combat crew.*

Psychiatric exam: The patient tells the story and describes the symptoms mentioned in the history. He has good insight into the fact that he is emotionally upset and says that the symptoms are beyond his control ... says he does not believe he can go up in a plane again. He seems sincere and straight forward and is very cooperative. He would like to do gunnery instructing without any flying being involved. In telling the story the patient had a noticeable tremor of the hands and several times seemed on the verge of tears when talking of his comrades killed in the crash. There were no psychotic symptoms present.[20]

Again we see the importance of the loss of this man's closest comrades, including in his case his whole original flight crew, in the development of his clinical picture. Losing those you love most makes you much more likely to break down in combat. The motivation to continue is just not as strong. After several more missions with significant additional trauma, he was finally ordered to get medical help. He was temporarily assigned to ground duty. We also see the similarity of his symptoms to those of the previous case.

Case three: 2nd Lieutenant, Pilot, B-17, Age 24
Chief Complaint: "Cannot Sleep"
Present Illness: This officer arrived in the ETO in May 1943 and has completed 18 missions. His first mission went to St. Nazaire where the flak was very heavy and he saw three B-17's go down. The next mission's target was Wilhelmshaven and the third Bremen; every ship in his group was hit by flak at Bremen but no ships were lost and no fighters encountered. On these trips he acted as co-pilot. Subsequent raids were carried to Huls, Hamburg, Paris, on all of which fighter opposition numbered in the hundreds. At St. Nazaire three bursts of flak hit his ship directly and one killed the navigator. The next raid to Paris was relatively easy. On the way home from an abortive trip to Hanover, his group was attacked by Hermann Goering's "Yellow Noses." Though no ships were lost, the squadron was severely shot up. The group performed such brilliant evasive action that the leader received the Silver Star. After this mission he commenced to worry seriously about missions, to sleep poorly. The last two raids were directed against Hanover and Kassel, again flak and fighter opposition were heavy, but he cannot clearly recollect details of this raid. For the past three weeks he has been sleeping about an hour or two a night even with the assistance of sleeping pills. On the night before a raid, he dreams of lines of "fighters coming in", and vivid bursts of flak. On the last few missions, he states

he has seen fighters that actually were not there. He has been feeling more and more tired, and took Benzedrine [the stimulant amphetamine] *before the last two raids. He was grounded when he asked for more Benzedrine, slept 18 hours, was then sent to the Hospital for narcosis treatment* [The flyers were put into a near coma-like sleep for up to 72 hours using high potency barbiturates.]. *He now feels very tired, ready for a rest, has no immediate interest in the war, but is anxious to return to combat when he is better.*

Psychiatric Examination: The officer is tense, tired and preoccupied with ideas of fighter opposition. His stream of talk is profuse once started, although he is somewhat retarded and depressed at present. The content of his thought is almost entirely concerned with combat and is so fixed that he cannot rid himself of visions of fighter planes during combat, but he realizes that these are illusions. He is excessively tired and believes he could sleep for a week. Fear of combat doesn't concern him. He is decisive in saying he wants to return to combat as soon as he's well. His sense of obligation to his crew is intense; sometimes he feels inadequate to meeting the emergencies that may turn up in combat despite his realization that he is well trained and the confidence that he's a good pilot. This feeling troubles him when he recalls that he, as pilot, is responsible for the other members of his crew.

Treatment: The patient received 72 hours of narcosis therapy, was much improved, and spent the following week at a Rest Home [These were quiet places where the men played cards and physical games and rested.]. *At the conclusion of this time, he said he felt completely well, was grateful for the treatment he had received, and asked to go back on a combat status. He was returned to his unit as "Operational Fatigue, recovered."*

Follow-up: The officer has completed 6 more combat missions since leaving the hospital and stated that he feels well except for "sweating out" his last (25th) mission which will complete the operational tour of duty.[21]

I marvel that a man can go through what this man did and want to keep flying with his men. What is even more remarkable is that his case is the norm rather than the exception. He appears to care more for his men than his own survival. He has no intention of abandoning them.

These cases paint the full spectrum of acute PTSD symptoms that combatants and ex-combatants struggle with, including disturbed sleep and subsequent exhaustion, nightmares, anxiety, intrusive thoughts and flashbacks (re-experiencing the trauma as if it was happening now). It is evident how important their comrades were to them and how much they cared for them. In the first and second cases the flyers did not start to break down until they had lost their closest comrades and friends. In the last case the pilot's devotion to his crew brought him quickly back to share the dangers of war with them.

These three authors (Hastings, Wright and Glueck) focused on trying to predict what would cause some men to break down in combat where others wouldn't. They explored the combatants' upbringing and their pre-military experiences but in the end were unable to find any predictable pattern. The high school standout was no more predisposed to success in weathering the trauma of combat than the dropout. Men from nontraditional homes did no worse than those from traditional ones. The quiet mouse was just as durable as the sports star.

Finally they looked at 150 consecutive men who were being sent home after completing their 25 combat missions and who had never appeared before the Central Medical Board for evaluation.[22] They found that they were just as symptomatic as those they had been treating in their hospitals, rest homes and clinics! Of the 150 men, 40 per cent were officers and 60 per cent enlisted men. Sixty-three per cent were less than 24-years old and 79 per cent single. Thirty-five per cent had been wounded or had bailed out, ditched (went down in water) or crashed – many multiple times. Over 80 per cent had been in severely damaged ships, or in which crewmen were wounded or killed, or had been badly lost over enemy territory.[23] One hundred per cent experienced fear and tension in relation to combat. The tension was most troubling before missions and especially before the last few missions, although as the authors noted, "Virtually all stated that they were relieved of tension by actual combat, no matter how dangerous or difficult it was."[24]

Of the 150 men interviewed who had successfully completed their 25 missions 95 per cent had diagnosable "operational fatigue" and 34 per cent had it severely, 39 per cent had insomnia and 79 per cent severe irritability. (This was defined as outbursts of anger and violence.) Also 22 per cent were unable to concentrate and 37 per cent were definitely depressed for long periods, 21 per cent were quite "seclusive," 45 per cent showed markedly increased alcohol use, and 29 per cent had developed a deep personal hatred toward the enemy.[25]

In other words, these psychiatrists found that those who had completed their 25 combat missions and were headed home had experienced the same types of trauma, faced the same fear and developed the same symptoms but had somehow not broken down and presented for medical attention. Why? These three psychiatrists did not answer this question; but two psychiatrists doing the same work with the infantry at the same time on another continent also asked this question and suggested some answers.

In North Africa in 1942–43 the US Army faced the German Army for the first time in WWII. The American troops had no combat experience. The

German Africa Corps was composed of seasoned veterans. The Germans had superior tanks in every respect but speed. They made fun of the American Sherman tank, calling it the "Ronson" after their cigarette lighter because it burst into flames whenever it was hit. One captured German exclaimed:

> Ronsons, you know ... Ronsons, yes, like for a cigarette. Our gunners see your tanks coming, all running over with that gasoline, and they say to each other, "Here comes another Ronson." Why do the Americans do this for us? Bang! And it burns like 20 haystacks. All the people in, my God ... Those funny tanks with the little guns, and so high and straight we can see them from a long way in our gunsights. Those square sides, and thin, the armor. We know if we hit one it goes up.[26]

Most German tanks had frontal armor nearly impervious to the 75mm cannon on the Sherman, and the Sherman's only advantage was its speed.[27] In a tank battle we generally needed a significant advantage in numbers of tanks to have a chance of winning.

In North Africa we had not yet developed full air superiority and the effective use of air support for ground combat that would lead to victory over the *Wehrmacht* in France. The Germans had the best machine gun with the most rapid, accurate fire, the MP-42. They also had the best single artillery piece of the war, their 88mm cannon (referred to by the Americans as simply "the 88").[28,29,30] The "88" had such high velocity that it could fire like a rifle and kill a soldier before he ever heard it. It could easily destroy any armored vehicle we had. Initially the American Army suffered serious losses and several defeats in North Africa.

The British started cheekily referring to the Americans as "our Italians," referring to their perception that Italian troops more easily succumbed to fear and ran, abandoning their German allies on the battlefield. Psychiatric casualties among the American troops were initially quite high.

Two American psychiatrists, Lt. Col. Roy R. Grinker and Maj. John P. Spiegel, were among those treating these casualties. They reported on their experiences in a small volume entitled *War Neuroses* published in 1945 but written and distributed to military medical officers in 1943.[31] Their book primarily describes their treatment of psychiatric casualties. In many instances they treated men who had lost their closest buddies, their flight crews or even most of the men of their company. The great majority of combatants never broke down but continued to fight in grim circumstances day after day. In their last chapter the authors finally state, "It would seem to be a more rational question to ask why the soldier does not succumb to anxiety, rather than why he does."[32] They suggested one reason and hinted at other reasons why men did not break down despite severe and prolonged combat. The veterans I have treated have consistently confirmed that these are the reasons most soldiers keep fighting effectively:

1 Identification with the group. "The soldier fights for his buddies." The group "becomes the object of considerable love and affection on the part of its members."[33] My vets over the years have constantly reiterated that love, affection and loyalty for their comrades are the only things that kept most combatants going.

Of lesser importance are:

2 Fighting for a clear objective as articulated by trusted officers. Most of the men I have treated were willing to follow any good officer who was leading them personally into combat. This is not Eisenhower encouraging the troops to liberate Fortress Europe. This is their company or platoon commander, who has fought with them from the beginning and has earned their respect and trust, saying, "This is what we have to do today," and then leading them to do it. It is closely tied to number one.
3 "But it won't happen to me; it may happen to others – but not to me."[34] This is that type of thinking to which the young are prone, that they are somehow invulnerable to the things that are hurting and killing everyone else. This youthful attitude is represented by a personalized license plate I recently saw on the back of a sports car driven by a teenager as it roared past me: "IMMORTAL."
4 Strong conscious hostility. "Only when the ego has been weakened by fatigue, deteriorated morale, or overwhelming catastrophe is the reaction of hostility replaced by one of crippling anxiety ..."[35] Although many finally break down from grief when all their closest comrades are killed, I have treated some that were instead consumed by such a desire for revenge they appeared to have lost their fear of death. Often they just want to kill until they are killed.

One of my Vietnam vets was in the state of "strong conscious hostility." He used to sleep with an armed grenade (safety pin removed) in his right hand underneath his chest. His justification for doing this was, "Just in case the gooks ever killed me, I would get a few of them too, when my hand released its grip." Needless to say, no one shared a foxhole with him.

Finally his commander ordered him to the rear even though he was a fearless soldier. If these "avengers" were not killed, sooner or later they were sent out of the unit because they were too dangerous, took too many risks, and in so doing jeopardized others. Sometimes they would rather kill than obey orders. Not many survive war.

Grinker and Spiegel found that breakdown in combat can occur quickly if there is no strong group identification and bond, but for most of those who break down it is a long process. As one's buddies and comrades are killed, one loses the defense of invulnerability. Reasoning goes like this: "Bill was killed. Bill was just like me – almost a part of me; therefore I will be killed too." There is often a corollary thought: "I'm glad it was Bill and not me." But this thought produces guilt and often further deterioration and misery.[36] The authors further conclude:

> Yet illness does not overtake the individual until all the above mentioned devices fail; and large numbers of soldiers subjected to the same intensity of stimulus never fall ill. In those who do succumb, in the largest number of cases, the ego has resisted for long periods of time. It is seldom the initial trauma, but usually a long chain of events, which lead to the appearance of symptoms.[37] [They add] ... The sight of friends injured and killed, the intense grief over the loss of good buddies, have a powerfully destructive effect on individual resistance. Repeatedly we have heard the statement, "I was all right until they killed my buddy."[38]

Certainly as the killing mounts, the transient defense of invulnerability evaporates. Each experienced combatant knows he can be killed and often recognizes the probability that he will be killed. Almost all just accept these facts and keep fighting.

The burden of grief also begins to mount.[39,40] At some point men have lost so many of those most dear to them that they can lose the will to continue to defend themselves. With continued fighting and constant sleep deprivation they can reach levels of grief and exhaustion where they "break." In one fashion or another they can no longer function effectively as soldiers. Combatants have used the phrase, "the 1000 yard stare," or for the very worst cases, "the 2000 yard stare" to describe the facial expression of men in this condition. One artist, Tom Lea, captured this state of mind in a combatant at Pelelieu in WWII. The artist described the scene he painted with these words: "I noticed a tattered Marine standing quietly by a corpsman, staring stiffly at nothing. His mind had crumbled in battle, his jaw hung, and his eyes were like two black empty holes in his head."[41] [Figure 2.11]

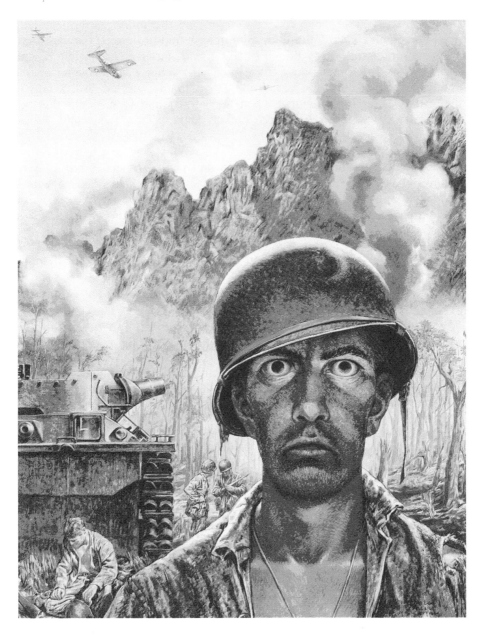

Figure 2.11 *Marines Call It That 2000 Yard Stare*

Does love and group cohesiveness provide the inner strength to help most combatants keep fighting despite intense and prolonged combat? As I pondered this issue, many things I had noticed started to come into clearer focus. Most of the men I have treated over the years went through horrible combat experiences but never broke down in the service. According to them, they actually got worse when they got home. How could that be? The pressure was off. They were out of danger. They were safe. It just didn't make sense to me. Now I had a reason why. They were parted from the "family" they loved most.

I can put it in simple terms. Say you and your extended family – your siblings, parents, grandparents, aunts, uncles and cousins all became a combat infantry unit. If it were a small family you would be a squad, a medium-sized family a platoon, and a large extended family a whole company of 200 or so. Now you are fighting for your lives against a merciless enemy. It is kill or be killed. There is no retreat to safety. How do you feel if you are sent home and your family is left there to fight, suffer and die?

E.B. Sledge in his autobiography *With The Old Breed* describes his experiences with the 1st Marine Division on Pelelieu and Okinawa in WWII. While in combat on Okinawa, he was puzzled by letters from men in their company who had been discharged home:

> Their early letters expressed relief over being back with family or with "wine, women, and song." But later the letters often became disturbingly bitter and filled with disillusionment. Some expressed a desire to return if they could get back into the old battalion. Considering the dangers and hardships those men had been through before they were sent home, and considering our situation in front of Shuri, the attitudes of our buddies who had returned Stateside puzzled us ... They expressed themselves in various ways, but the gist of their disillusionment was a feeling of alienation from everyone but their old comrades ... all the good life and luxury didn't seem to take the place of old friendships forged in combat.[42]

Being "in front of Shuri" on Okinawa was probably the most dangerous place on the planet at that time. The men at home who wanted to return had probably already been through Guadalcanal, Cape Gloucester and Pelelieu. The 1st Marine Division suffered well over 100 per cent casualties by the end of the war. The willingness of these Marines to return and face combat with their buddies illustrates how strong the bond was that bound them to their fellow combatants. Certainly it was stronger than their fear of death.

A fighter pilot who saw extensive combat against the Japanese during WWII described his relationship with his fellow pilots in these words: "... Several of them were to become as close as brothers to me with that special camaraderie generated in combat by the unspoken but understood commitment to risk our lives for each other ..."[43]

One Marine rifleman described the bond between himself and his closest buddies in these terms: "... In war, loyalties shrink down past country and family to one or two men who will be with you. They become more important than anyone else in the world, more precious than father and mother, sister and brother, wife and girl ..."[44] If our beloved family members (or comrades even closer than family) are in danger, most of us cannot simply abandon them and go to safety. These comments are from an infantryman who had been wounded at Anzio in 1944 and evacuated to safety:

> We were taken off the beachhead and sent to a hospital in Naples and got sewed up. Several weeks later we were all down at the hospital – lots of us down there in Naples. One of the officers of the 504th [A unit trapped at the Anzio beachhead under constant German shelling] came down and said, "Anyone from the 504th who can stand up, can walk, meet me down here at the end of the hall." We all went down, about 40 of us in casts, bandages, arms in slings and everything. He said, "Your buddies up there are catching hell and we're looking for volunteers." We said, "Hell, we'll go." We just had the best-spirited bunch of scrappers you ever saw. I was wearing a kind of diaper. And the nurse gave me a bottle of boric acid soap to keep it (my wound) clean with. We went; only one guy didn't go.[45]

Despite their wounds 39 of 40 hospitalized men returned to combat to support their comrades in the murderous hell that was Anzio! Fear shrinks in the face of a soldier's love for his comrades.

One combatant who led a company in Korea and battalions and brigades in Vietnam put it very directly:

> Another and far more transcendent love came to us unbidden on the battlefields, as it does on every battlefield in every war man has ever fought. We discovered in that depressing, hellish place, where death was our constant companion, that we loved each other. We killed for each other, we died for each other, and we wept for each other. And in time we came to love each other as brothers.[46]

The bottom line is that units without that type of love for each other, that "esprit de corps" or unit solidarity, do not fight well. They do not win. They run.

Richard Waller was a professor at Columbia University and a World War I veteran when he wrote the book *The Veteran Comes Back* in 1944, trying to prepare the public for the return of the WWII vets. Speaking about the essential fidelity and care soldiers develop for their comrades in arms, he notes, "Some solidarity, however, must remain, or the war must stop. For when people lose the sense of solidarity, they also lose the will to fight."[47]

Many of my infantry veterans who killed only did it because the alternative was to let their beloved war family be killed. Like Arly, who believed he was the only man in his squad who would kill the enemy, they protected the other men they loved. Those who killed as a unit (aircrews and shipmates) usually did it from afar as a team. Sometimes they were able initially to do it only because they were not able to see the humans they were killing. They could pretend they were just sinking a ship, destroying a tank or bombing a factory building. But eventually they would have to face the full impact and responsibility entailed in destroying those war machines and buildings and maiming and killing the men and women inside.

Here, then, we have the two forces for beginning and continuing war. It starts with one side, often led by a ruthless tyrant or guided by a philosophy that makes enemies less than truly human, seeing the other side as a threat that will not give them what they want through peaceful negotiation. Through the medium of racist propaganda, the demonizing begins. "They have besmirched our holy soil. They are choking off our economic lifeblood. They are destroying our freedoms and revered way of life." They frighten the opposing tribe, nation, or people, who begin their own response that starts to demonize the aggressor. Actions and reactions lead to some killing, and the propaganda and demonizing intensify. Military units are formed, and that great human power of working together in loving teams is activated. The serious fighting begins, and it is so horrible that only love, stronger than the fear of death and the loathing of killing, can keep it going and take it to its conclusion. And the cost is terrible for the men and women who shoulder the burden of the fighting and killing.

Notes

1   Grossman, Lt. Col. Dave, *On Killing*, pp. 3–4.
2   Lorenz, Conrad, *On Aggression*, p. 44.
3   Ibid pp. 81–103.

4   Ibid pp. 23–6.

5   Ibid pp. 35–6.

6   Rhodes, Anthony, *Propaganda: The Art of Persuasion: World War II*, pp. 59, 48, 196. Figures 2.3 and 2.4 in text are courtesy of the US Library of Congress.

7   Ibid p. 45. Figure 2.5 in text is courtesy of the US Library of Congress.

8   Ibid pp. 92–3, 96.

9   Ibid pp. 262, 252.

10 Ibid pp. 261, 175. Figure 2.6 in text is courtesy of the US National Archives.

11 Ibid pp. 168, 170–1. Figure 2.7 in text is courtesy of the US National Archives.

12 Ibid pp. 226, 175, 169. Figure 2.8 in text is courtesy of the US Library of Congress. Figures 2.9 and 2.10 in text are courtesy of the US National Archives.

13 Allen, Thomas B. and Norman Polmar, *Code-Name Downfall*, pp. 291–4 explore the same issues. The following articles continue that debate and strongly suggest that far more lives were spared because the A-bombs were used than the A-bombs killed. "Remembrances of the War and the Bomb" by Taro Takemi, MD, *JAMA*, Aug 5, 1983 – Vol. 250, No. 5, pp. 618–19; "Dr. Takemi and the Atomic Bomb" by Daniel T. Cloud, MD, *JAMA*, Aug 2, 1995 – Vol. 274, No. 5, pp. 413–15; "Invasion Most Costly" by Norman Polmar and Thomas B. Allen, *U.S. Naval Proceedings* 121, No. 8, Aug. 1995, pp. 51–6.

14 Lord, Walter, *Incredible Victory*, p. 242, a second pilot reacted in a similar way.

15 Davis, Russell, *Marine at War*, pp. 231–4.

16 Hastings, Major Donald W., Captain David C. Wright, and Captain Bernard C. Glueck, *Psychiatric Experiences of the Eighth Air Force: First Year of Combat (July 4, 1942– July 4, 1943)* pp. 13–19. One of the psychiatrists went on a bombing mission deep into Germany with an experienced crew and saw what they went through first hand. This is his description of the crew, the mission, and how they coped:

> A brief exposition of the circumstances surrounding the making of these observations is necessary. The airplane, a B-17, on a mission over a distant target in enemy-occupied Europe, had most of its controls shot out by attacking planes before reaching the target, so that the ship was knocked out of formation. The pilot, however, with the exercise of great skill and strength, persisted in making an effective bomb run. Following this the lone airplane was attacked by about 100 FW 190 fighters over a period of perhaps three-quarters of an hour, during which time extraordinary damage was done to the plane and crew. Virtually all the crew were wounded, three severely, and one became anoxic as a result of the simultaneous stunning explosion of a 20mm cannon shell next to him, and the severance of his oxygen system. Almost all of the control cables were cut in various places, the oxygen, hydraulic, and electrical systems were knocked out, the interphone and radio systems destroyed, a small fire started in the bomb-bay, large holes were put through both wings, holes were in two propellers, bomb-bay, fuselage and nose; the tail assembly received so many direct cannon hits that it vibrated violently and, after inspection by the flight engineer, was expected to tear off entirely at any moment. Following the cessation of the fighter attack, therefore, the crew did not expect that the ship would successfully cross the channel, that a smooth ditching would be possible, or that in the event the English coast were reached an uneventful landing could be effected. In almost any eventuality attempts to take care of the severely wounded men would have strongly prejudiced the chances of survival of the rest. Such were the circumstances. The personalities involved varied greatly. The pilot was big, easy-going, emotionally stable but unaggressive, essentially introverted, and extremely intelligent. The co-pilot was a

tightly-wound, aggressive cyclothyme, with a clear history of a previous mixed manic-depressive attack of disabling degree. The navigator was a quiet, rigid, but fundamentally well-balanced person. The bombardier was a vigorous, fast thinking extrovert, irritable and outspoken. The radio operator does not come within the bounds of this discussion, having been unconscious or disoriented from anoxia during most of the period. The top turret gunner-engineer was an energetic, over-compensating extrovert, independent and uninhibited to the point of eccentricity. The ball turret gunner was a small, quiet and self-sufficient introvert, cool, impersonal, and emotionally tough. The right waist gunner was markedly extroverted, merry, careless of consequences, of opinion, of the past or of the future. The left waist gunner was a rather seclusive, shy, infinitely conscientious introvert, who never drank, never smoked, never let himself go at all. The tail gunner was basically rigid, limited and simple in imagination and outlook, completely thorough and dependable.

Such schematically were the personalities. The reactions of the men were remarkably *alike*. During the violent combat and in the acute emergencies that arose during it they were all quietly precise on the interphone and split-second decisive in action. The tail gunner, right waist gunner, and navigator were severely wounded early in the fight, but all three kept at their duties efficiently and without cessation until the combat was over, their guns were destroyed, or, in the case of the navigator the home station was in sight. The burden of the emergency work with controls, oxygen, wounded men, and reparable battle damage fell on the pilot, engineer, ball turret gunner, and the left waist gunner, and all four functioned with rapidity, skilful effectiveness, and with no lost motion. The burden of decisions during and particularly after the combat, rested essentially on the pilot, and in secondary details on the co-pilot and the bombardier. The decisions were arrived at with care and with speed, were unquestioned once they had been made, and proved excellent. In the period over the channel and over England when disaster was momentarily expected, the alternative plans of action were made clearly and with no thought other than for the safety of the entire crew. All, at this period, were quiet, unobtrusively cheerful, and ready for anything.

There was at no time paralysis, panic, unclear thinking, faulty or confused judgement, or self-seeking, in any of these men.

It was striking that the emergency did not tend to increase the difference in the reaction patterns of the differing personalities; rather they came to act in much more similar fashion than usual. One could not possibly have inferred from their behavior that this one was an unstable cyclothyme and that one was a shy quiet introspective man. They all became outwardly calm, precise in thought, and rapid in action.

17   Allen op. cit. p. 77.
18   Ethell, Jeffrey and Alfred Price, *One Day in a Long War*, pp. 190–2.
19   Hastings op. cit. pp. 289–300.
20   Ibid pp. 241–51.
21   Ibid pp. 301–7.
22   Ibid pp. 113–56.
23   Ibid pp. 132–3.
24   Ibid pp. 143–4.
25   Ibid pp. 134–6.
26   Phibbs, Brendan, *The Other Side of Time*, pp. 75–6.
27   Ibid pp. 74–5.
28   Collins, Brig. Gen. James L. and Lt. Col. Eddy Bauer, *The Marshall Cavendish Illustrated Encyclopedia of World War II*, Vol. 12, p. 1655. The author notes about the

Tiger pictured, "Undisputed master of the first tank battles in Normandy: the Tiger with all its earlier teething troubles eliminated. In the hands of a master Panzer technician like ... Wittman, the Tiger was a deadly weapon. In a classic battle Wittman's solitary Tiger knocked out 25 British tanks within minutes."

29 Heiferman, Ronald, *World War II*, p. 156, German 88mm cannon in North Africa.
30 MacDonald, Charles B., *Company Commander*, p. 118, Sherman tank with its "high silhouette."
31 Grinker, Roy R. and John P. Spiegel, *War Neuroses*.
32 Ibid p. 115.
33 Ibid pp. 117–18.
34 Ibid p. 120.
35 Ibid pp. 60, 120.
36 Ibid p. 122.
37 Ibid p. 123.
38 Ibid p. 69.
39 Smith, S.E., editor, *The United States Marine Corps in World War II*. These black and white photos give some idea of the grim fighting in the Pacific.
40 Steinberg, Rafael, *Island Fighting*, pp. 184–91, Combat at Pelelieu. Paintings by Tom Lea.
41 Ibid p. 187. Tom Lea's painting and comments from Pelelieu.
42 Sledge, E.B., *With the Old Breed*, pp. 272–3.
43 Lopez op. cit. p. 54.
44 Davis op. cit. p. 12.
45 O'Donnell, Patrick, *Beyond Valor*, p. 88.
46 Moore, Lt. Gen. Harold, G. and Joseph L. Galloway, *We were Soldiers Once ... and Young*, p. xviii.
47 Waller, Richard, *The Veteran Comes Back*, p. 37.

Chapter 3

The Trauma of War and the Emotional Cost to the Common Men Who Fight It

I first began treating VA patients in 1981. Ten years later, in 1991, I would have agreed with Tom Brokaw's 1998 assertion in *The Greatest Generation* that the WWII generation was somehow better than subsequent generations. I would have based that erroneous conclusion on my patient sample up to then.

In that first ten years of clinical work, I saw a lot of troubled Vietnam vets. These men were often combat vets with disturbed sleep and nightmares, daily intrusive thoughts of the war, and flashbacks (reliving the event in the here and now – like a nightmare while awake). They were almost always abusing drugs, alcohol or both. They often had psychiatric diagnoses in addition to PTSD, such as serious depression, psychosis or personality disorders. They were failing in their personal and work relationships. They tended to be spiritually lost, either disconnected from the Divine or blaming God. They externalized their problems, blaming others for their miseries, and coped poorly. They had lots of secondary medical problems, and – unless they responded to treatment – they often died at a younger age from medical or psychiatric causes.

On the other hand, the WWII and Korean War vets I was seeing looked very different. They were married, raising children and grandchildren, earning an effective living, making a difference in their communities, staying clean and sober and doing all this despite symptoms and memories from their wars. They had deep spiritual roots and took responsibility for their lives. They were the aging pillars of the community.

I now believe that this apparent generational difference in the soldiers I was treating was caused by a serious sampling error in my work. As the next decade (1991–2001) of my clinical work unfolded, I began seeing on an outpatient basis many of the vast majority of better-coping Vietnam vets. As I worked with this new (to me) group of Vietnam vets, the reasons for my initial sampling error – resulting in the false conclusion that the WWII and Korean generations were somehow "better" than the Vietnam generation – became clearer. These reasons included:

1   The least adaptive and most deeply disturbed of the WWII and Korean War survivors were dead before I started VA work in 1981. They had died young, just as I was seeing happen to the poorer functioning Vietnam vets.
2   The majority of the most adaptive Vietnam vets were not coming to the VA in 1981–91. They were out working and living life.
3   Many of the WWII and Korean War vets who seemed to be doing so well in 1981–91 had struggled terribly in their immediate post-war years. By the time I started seeing them later in their lives, they were doing much better. As I gained their trust and became more experienced and effective as a therapist, I began to realize that if I had seen them in 1951, they would have looked like the "poorer functioning" Vietnam vets I was seeing in 1981.
4   I began seeing the fruits of our therapeutic efforts as many of the initially poorly coping Vietnam vets responded to treatment and other healing life events and started coping much better. By 1995 both these "recovering" Vietnam vets and the Vietnam vets who were seeking treatment for the first time started to look just like the better functioning WWII and Korean War vets I was already treating.

Remember that Drs. Hastings, Wright and Glueck, in their work with those who developed "operational fatigue" (their term for acute battlefield PTSD) in the 8th US Air Force in 1942–43, had hypothesized that the reason some broke down while others did not might have been due to their pre-military adaptations and experiences. They theorized that those with poorer pre-military coping skills and upbringing might be more prone to break down in combat. They looked for this but did not find it.

Pre-military experience and adaptive strengths did not seem to predict who would break down and who wouldn't in the combat setting, but it is important to note that the doctors did not attempt to predict how these men would cope when they returned home to civilian life. When that happened, their pre-military experiences and adaptive strengths would become important. The power of group solidarity, the love of comrades forged in the life-and-death crucible of combat, the binding and saving esprit de corps – these factors kept the weak as well as the strong integrated enough that most were able to keep fighting effectively. This integrating force was lost on repatriation.

Released from military life and the supportive brotherhood of their combat unit, the previously more troubled men did have more difficulty coping on their own after their discharge. Those with a propensity for alcohol or drug abuse, with the added stress of PTSD, now had real trouble without the discipline and group cohesiveness of the military to keep them in line. Those with a propensity for depression and psychosis found it exacerbated by the sleep deprivation and the heightened arousal that are natural symptoms of PTSD; and if they drank or abused drugs, their vulnerability to other psychiatric problems was further exacerbated. If they were spiritually disconnected or the families they returned to were poorly functioning, they naturally had less support to help them reintegrate and positively cope with civilian life.

By 1995 my Vietnam vets who responded to treatment were looking more and more like the surviving WWII and Korean War vets. About this same time, I started seeing more of the large majority of originally better coping Vietnam vets. They came in as new grandfathers, successful businessmen and professionals, seeking initial treatment for problems with PTSD that had "just never gone away" or had been reactivated by current life stressors. These Vietnam vets looked like the very successful copers of the "greatest generation" I was already treating.

Several years ago the topic of alcohol abuse came up in my two WWII/ Korea PTSD groups, which also included three men who had served in both Korea and Vietnam. Of the 25 men combined in both groups at that time, twenty had suffered from severe alcohol abuse for several years after the war. The important distinction was that they had stopped and were therefore still alive and coping much better than when they had been drinking. One WWII vet in the group returned to alcohol abuse and died while intoxicated a few years later.

The typical pattern of how war affects the lives of most vets who have served extensively in combat is the same, whether they served in WWII, Korea, Vietnam or any other war. In this chapter I will present the basic symptoms most combatants struggle with and the types of experiences that engendered these symptoms. First, the vast majority of soldiers get through their war experiences without breaking down or receiving psychiatric treatment. But, just as the psychiatrists found in the 8th Air Force in 1942–43, the men who weren't treated had the same symptoms as the men who came to psychiatric attention with acute PTSD in the service.

Remember, of the 150 men who had completed their 25 combat bombing missions and were headed home, "95 per cent had operational fatigue." My experience with my patients supports this. They come home, and for the next several years they have battle dreams almost every night. They experience intrusive thoughts of the war on a daily basis. In the right circumstances they suffer flashbacks. They are hyper-alert and very sensitive to loud noises, war-associated sounds and smells and other individually specific stimuli. They often have little tolerance for anything that reminds them of their former enemy.

Despite this, they are tough and adaptable and in some ways very confident. They may worry they are "cracking up," but they don't. They keep moving ahead in life. Most don't seek treatment in this phase. They are young and strong. They have survived some of the worst life has to offer, and deep down they know it. They usually do not talk about what they have been through. After a few years the acute symptoms start to abate in intensity and frequency. They become thoroughly involved in their civilian activities. People who knew them before the war see definite changes, but after several years no one else, except their wives, would really know they were combat vets.

The PTSD symptoms rarely disappear completely. Around the anniversary of certain war events, more symptoms appear. For Vietnam vets this is often the New Year because of the Tet offensives regularly launched by the Vietcong and North Vietnamese. Other dates are much more group – or person – specific. For JR, mentioned in Chapter 2, April and May are difficult because late April was when his crewmembers were killed and wounded and he was wounded on his last mission. For Hank it is December 7, when the Japanese attacked his ship at Pearl Harbor. For Tim, a medic with the 1st Infantry Division, it is June because of the Normandy invasion and D-Day. I am convinced that the brain has an uncanny means of tracking dates. This may have a survival advantage, putting veterans "on alert," prepared to fight the battle over again at this specific time of this year too, if necessary. Almost all combat vets experience this "anniversary reaction" to some degree.

Vets will be doing fine on the surface for years, but events can occur that trigger problems. The Persian Gulf War reactivated symptoms in most vets. The current terrorist war that flared starting with the attacks on the World Trade Center and the Pentagon on September 11, 2001 has had the same effect. In these instances the battle dreams become more frequent, as do the intrusive thoughts and flashbacks. Hyper-alertness becomes more problematic. Unfortunately we seem to be in a time of constant war and threats of war, and the only relief for some vets is to limit their media exposure.

The death or illness of a close family member can reactivate war-related symptoms. It is too much like that previous horrible pain of losing beloved comrades in battle. Being hospitalized for the first time since being wounded in war often reawakens symptoms. Being actively involved in the present is one of the better ways of driving the symptoms away. Retirement, with its fewer demands on the here and now, often provides an opportunity for the symptoms to return.

Most vets hate to get angry and try to avoid it as they mature. Anger is closely linked with too many of their combat experiences and can trigger intrusive war thoughts and feelings. They also know that they have the ability to kill. Ex-infantrymen in particular detest having someone approach them from behind or surprise them. They can respond automatically with potentially lethal moves when surprised, and this conditioned response can last their whole lives.

One of my WWII combat vets served in the Philippines as an infiltrator, killing men with a piano wire garrote and a knife. He was hospitalized after being rescued from a POW camp, where, he joked, he had been a "guest of ithe Japs" for three years. While hospitalized the following occurred:

> I was sleeping in a hospital bed when a little nurse walked up quietly and touched my head. The next thing I knew, I had grabbed her by the nose and mouth, ripped her head back, and was bringing my knee down to break her spine when I noticed her hair. It was blond. I was just able to stop in time. If her hair had been black, she would be dead. Luckily I had never killed anyone with blond hair, and I knew something was wrong. I was sick about what I almost did and felt so bad for the terror I caused her.

A combat infantryman I had seen occasionally for years, providing him medication to help him sleep, came to see me quite disturbed. He had a large, strong son who was an outstanding high school wrestler. His son had initiated a wrestling match with him, despite his dad's resistance, out of what appeared to be a desire to feel a little closer to his "old man." The patient reported, "I'm not quite sure what happened. He nearly had me pinned when the next instant I had him in a lethal chokehold. My wife was slapping my face, screaming for me to stop. Thank God she happened to be there! I could have killed him." His son had put him in such a vulnerable position that an automatic combat reflex was triggered. He acted before he consciously thought. We processed this in detail. The bottom line was he could not let himself get in a position where he felt threatened to this degree. His son learned a hard lesson. He found out why his dad had never wrestled with him "like other dads did with their sons." He was protecting them both from an experience like this.

It would be a serious error to imagine from these last two examples that combat vets have control problems or are prone to violence. This is supported by the fact that the incarceration rate for veterans is less than half that of adult male non-veterans in federal and state prisons in the United States and the homicide rate for the civilian black male population is twelve times higher than for black males in the US Army.[1,2] Unless they are drunk, ex-combatants have the tightest emotional and behavioral control of any group I have ever treated. They developed this control in the crucible of combat, and for some, in POW camps. I have treated many ex-POWs over the years. They were often beaten, starved, mocked and humiliated by their captors. If they lost control in the face of this or even showed emotion, the consequences could be much worse, as their guards would only increase the level of abuse. These men could be seething inside with rage and never act on it or show a flicker of emotion. Combat vets learn to face seemingly incapacitating fear and continue to think and act clearly. Through these experiences they develop what at times appears to be almost super-human emotional control. The automatic responses of self-preservation, illustrated by the reaction of the vets in the two stories above, are simply faster than thought. They are learned, reflexive responses that kept them alive in combat.

There are many other automatic responses. Most vets will be uncomfortable in crowds. "It is just not safe to bunch up. You are too vulnerable and inviting a target to artillery or automatic weapons." And though the conscious thought is not there, years later the automatic emotional response remains. Do not expect most combat vets to be comfortable sitting in the middle of a restaurant. Most need a spot in a corner where they can see the windows and doors, with a strong wall to their backs. They may not have the conscious thought, but the emotional response remains.

Most combat vets dislike gunfire, and, in my experience, many stop hunting, but they usually will not give up their personal weapons. Most of my WWII vets keep a weapon nearby while trying to sleep; some still keep one under the pillow, some in a drawer in the nightstand, but always close enough to have ready access. It is a wartime habit that is almost impossible to break in the current climate of media violence and reported crime. I had thought that years of therapy might have changed this, but as we talked about it in a recent group session, I learned that all but one man in the group still had weapons nearby at night.

For most combatants it is a lot harder to get close to others after the war. The violent loss of beloved comrades produces a resistance to "ever getting that close again." To fight successfully as a team, they have to become deeply trusting and bonded to one another. The inevitable death of many of their fellow combatants pains them deeply. This is part of the price of participating in a strong combat unit. The survivors are instinctively reluctant to make themselves that vulnerable again by loving deeply. Often this does not become explicitly conscious but operates on an unconscious level, partially blocking their attempts at deeper intimacy.

There is another thought that keeps vets cautious in their relationships, and that is some version of the question, "If I really told them what I have done, what would they think of me?" There are combat memories hidden in the deepest corners of their minds that they don't want to think about. They are very reluctant to share these memories with others because of what it might mean about what they are or who other people might perceive them to be. Thinking of what they have participated in or done often brings up another question, "What type of man could do that?" Their answer is often self-condemning.

But enough of these generalizations. Let's look at more cases, for the truth is always clearer in the reality of the details. These cases, just like the general description of symptoms presented above, represent regular, war-related PTSD. They are not exceptional. I present them to help the reader who has not experienced combat develop some deeper understanding of what ordinary men face in combat and in their subsequent lives.

Norm's combat experiences started with the hell that was Tarawa. It was the first major US amphibious assault of the war on a tenaciously defended beach. The Japanese were ready; they fought to nearly the last man. The fighting was brutal and the carnage unimaginable, even to those who experienced it. Norm waded through surf that seemed more blood than water. It was a maelstrom of killing and maiming. He emptied the magazine of his BAR (Browning automatic rifle) into a Japanese officer just after the officer had decapitated one of Norm's friends with a samurai sword in a banzai charge.

After Tarawa Norm was selected to participate in a special mission. That mission involved military and civilian casualties, including children, as they were forced to destroy a weapons research facility that included a large apartment building. It still troubles him deeply, but because of the oath of secrecy he took as a mission participant, he feels he cannot talk about it publicly. He then participated in the end of the battle for Saipan, clearing Japanese from caves and bunkers as the island was being secured. He was preparing to help invade Japan when the atom bombs ended the war. He described his difficulties upon returning home:

> I tried college but I was too restless to sit through lectures, and I was having too many nightmares and intrusive thoughts of the war to successfully study. I was initially too broke to drink much. I finally got a good enough job to afford more liquor than was good for me. I started drinking to try to forget and sleep. I soon learned to stay away from everyone while drinking for fear I might hurt someone in a fight. I stayed sober just enough to do my job. For the most part I avoided people except at work. I was working at the Sun Valley Resort, and luckily the hours and working conditions were flexible or I probably wouldn't have kept the job. Then I met a woman at work and fell in love. She was very patient with me and marrying her was the best thing I ever did. It took 27 years, but I finally stopped drinking and joined her church. I saw what her religion did for her and our children. It helped them be better people, and I finally decided I needed that myself.

Norm never can enjoy a beach: "I see bodies rolling in the surf to this day. October and November are always bad because of Tarawa. I get more tense and edgy, don't go out much if I can help it, and stay away from the news." To this day the sight and sounds of little children – especially when they cry – remind him of the children unavoidably killed on the special mission he went on. "I think of what we did to them and their families. I wonder if I can ever feel truly forgiven for what I have done?"

Norm's PTSD symptoms were severely reactivated by the Oklahoma City bombing and the destruction of the World Trade Center in New York City. "It was too much like what we did in the war." He has grandchildren who are starting to have a third generation of crying babies. Those cries always bring him back to the thought of those killed during his secret mission. Norm went into treatment after he became more symptomatic because of failing health and retirement.

Ken was a mortarman in the 84th Infantry Division in Europe. He saw his first action attacking the Siegfried Line in the fall of 1944. A few months after the Battle of the Bulge, he was wounded in the right thigh by German mortars near the Roer River. He was hospitalized in Liege, and while he was there the hospital was hit by a German buzz bomb. It destroyed one whole wing – killing many of the wounded, and their nurses and physicians. In the spring of 1945 he returned to his unit as they approached the Elbe River and the German Army was collapsing. His division was on its way to help in the invasion of Japan when the atom bombs ended the war. Speaking of his return to Idaho after the war, Ken explains:

> After a few weeks me and a few of my friends and cousins realized we really weren't fit for civilized society yet. We were just too wild and dangerous. I worried that if I got mad I might just kill someone without hardly giving it a second thought. The five of us got together and pooled our money and got a boat to the Alaskan panhandle. We bought supplies and had a fisherman drop us off on an uninhabited island where we bivouacked, fished and hunted. The boat would come by once a month with additional supplies. We stayed there about a year. When we returned we had settled down enough to be safe to be around.

He went back to farming and has raised a family. He never talked about the war with his family, but they knew it still bothered him. After he retired he got sick and was seen at our hospital. The retirement and illness had reactivated his PTSD. A smart internist questioned him, discovered this and sent him to see me.

Ken has thrived in group therapy. He gave me a book to read about a company in his division, *The Men of Company K*. It is one of the best books I have read for helping a noncombatant understand what war is like.[3] My vets are always trying to make me a little better psychiatrist. Ken is a man of few words, but he told me of his difficulties getting close to people after the war:

> We trained together starting in 1942. Guys from all over the USA. You become close then but even more so when the action starts. By the time people start getting killed, you are like brothers, maybe even closer. It hurts real bad to lose them. You never want to make the mistake of getting close again. It makes it hard after the war.

Jim was a teenage seaman on the battleship *Mississippi*. "I lied about my age to get in because of Pearl Harbor." He served on the *Mississippi* throughout the South Pacific. He was there when she and five of the battleships sunk and later salvaged at Pearl Harbor got their revenge – helping sink a Japanese fleet at the Surigao Straits in the battle of Leyte

Gulf. "I saw those Japanese ships sink and all those men die, and even
though they were dirty Japs, it still hurt to know you helped do it." They
participated in many invasions and naval engagements. He was manning a
40mm anti-aircraft gun in the heat of a kamikaze attack off Okinawa, when
a crewman was decapitated in the excitement by "standing up in front of
our barrels." On another attack a kamikaze crashed near his gun. The pilot's
head with the helmet still on rolled right to his feet. "I picked it up and
threw it overboard."

After the war he returned to farming. He came into treatment at the
insistence of his wife. During the crop dusting seasons he would start
drinking. "Those stinking crop dusters always got me thinking and
dreaming about the war, and I would drink to try to sleep, and it would get
out of hand." He would have flashbacks and be convinced the low-flying
crop dusters were kamikazes; he would try to shoot them down with his
hunting rifle. His wife knew something had to be done. Group therapy and
alcohol treatment were helpful. But during Desert Storm he had two
grandchildren in the Navy and lost a grandson in a car accident near his
home. These events temporarily stirred up florid PTSD symptoms again.

Ted was a captain in charge of a mobile artillery unit in France and
Germany. He describes the painful burden he began to carry as the officer
in charge:

> I had to face the fact that I gave orders and people died. It sometimes seemed I
> was picking who would die by the assignments I ordered. I started to hate being
> in charge. We would shell the Germans in a French village. They would retreat
> and we would move in. There would be women and children that our shells had
> killed.

His unit was one of the first to get to the Remagen Bridge over the Rhine
in March 1945. They helped defend the bridge against intense German
counterattacks. He was nearby when the bridge finally collapsed ten
days after its capture – killing many men on the bridge. He lost men
near that bridge – men to whom he was "like a father." When he returned
to New York, he had his first panic attack trying to cross the Brooklyn
Bridge.

He had the usual several years of intense symptoms after the war, but
despite that he used the GI bill to complete college, become a successful
engineer, and raise a family. When he retired, his symptoms got worse and

he came in to get help because he could not get himself to cross a bridge without having a panic attack.

Joe was a scout in the 30th Infantry Division in Europe, a division that saw constant combat from Normandy to the end of the war in Europe. He was wounded in the head and face by direct fire from 88mm German cannons. Two weeks later he was back fighting with his company:

> We were engaged with a group of Germans in trenches on a slight rise. Under cover of our artillery fire we charged and were able get into their trenches and drive them out, capturing many of them. We made them get out of the trenches with their hands over their heads where we could see them clearly. Just then we were engulfed in a terrific artillery barrage – all 88mm, so we never heard it coming. We were somewhat protected in the trenches, but all the German prisoners were blown into pieces which rained down on us. I was completely covered by their body parts and blood. I hated their 88mm. Once my wife wanted to buy an Oldsmobile 88. I couldn't let her do it, nor tell her why. I never could have ridden in that car or even had it around. The word and number 88 still make me think of the war even now.

Joe loved the men in his squad and company. About a week before the war ended in Europe, they were moving across an open field toward a German town. To their left was a German autobahn:

> It was a road like one of our freeways now. I was in the lead and just as I was approaching the edge of the town a German Tiger tank came out from the underpass of the autobahn where it had been concealed. I fell flat on my face and it drove right by me. All the men in my squad were killed as it tore through us and the rest of the company, machine-gunning the men who were caught out in the open. It then clanked off into the woods. There was nothing we could do to stop it. Half the company was killed and wounded. How do you go on after that? It broke my heart to lose all those men just before the war ended.

Joe's post-war life followed the same pattern as so many others. He struggled with daily intrusive thoughts and nightmares for years. He took over his dad's shoe repair shop, married, and raised a family. He finally retired to a little farm. He was never comfortable driving on freeways and after he retired could not get himself to travel on them until he got some treatment. To this day there are two things that cause him to have flashbacks of German Tiger tanks. The first is fog. "The Germans would always counterattack with tanks in the fog because fog neutralized our airpower.

When it gets foggy at our home in the winter, it is just like being back in Europe, and I see tanks coming out of the woods." The second is the smell of diesel fumes. "Whenever I smell diesel, I start seeing Tigers out of the corner of my eyes." German tanks ran on diesel and American tanks on gasoline. Joe came to treatment because a trusted physician persuaded him to accept a referral to see me. "They never had a group like this for WWII vets at my previous VA. It has sure helped."

Jed was a sergeant in the 2nd Infantry Division in Korea. He served mainly as a forward artillery observer but was also a section leader (the artillery equivalent of a squad leader). His unit was vastly outnumbered by the Red Chinese when the Chinese crossed the Yalu River and began driving the American and UN forces back towards Seoul in the winter of 1950–1951. "Over those few months there always seemed to be thousands of them to our few hundreds."

He got very close to the men he served with and led. "It is impossible to express how deeply you felt about the men you fought with and how much their deaths hurt. I loved my parents and was very sad when they died, but it hurt me more to lose my comrades than to see my parents pass on." In February 1951, Jed's unit was nearly surrounded; they had to fight for their lives:

> I had just emptied two clips of ammo into a group of Chinese right in front of our trench, killing several, when a man near me suddenly stood, threw down his weapon, and raised his arms in surrender. Surrender was not in my vocabulary. I was ready to fight until I was killed. I nearly shot the man who surrendered, but many others were surrendering also. Instead, I turned and ran. As I did so, I took a slug through both lungs. The Chinese stripped me of my overcoat and boots and left me there to die as they rounded up the rest of the men who had surrendered. I am not sure how I lived through the night. My woolen underwear helped, but with the wound I had I should have died within a few hours, if not minutes. The next day an officer appeared. He had all the POWs who could walk sent back under guard towards China. A buddy, whose leg was shattered by a bullet, and I were dragged into a farmer's hut. I know they thought we would just die. I guess God had other plans.

Jed and his buddy lay neglected for a month in that hut just behind the Chinese lines near the 38th Parallel:

> The Chinese provided us no care or food. Occasionally we were beaten or kicked, and one of my ribs was broken during one of the beatings. But we

couldn't get away so we were not guarded very closely. A Korean farmer was being forced to cook for the Chinese soldiers. Each night he would bring us water and the burnt rice scraped from the pots he cooked with. That burnt rice tasted like candy! He risked his life for us. The Chinese would have killed him if they had ever caught him feeding us. I love him and owe him so much. How I would like to find him and thank him!

A month after Jed and his buddy's capture, they awoke to find the Chinese gone. The American unit that drove the Chinese away rescued them.

Jed was discharged home in 1952. He did day labor and ran machinery for local farmers for three years. "I was drinking heavily to try to sleep and forget the war, and I was going nowhere until I met my wife." Meeting her prompted him to "seek work with a future." He was hired as a civilian by the Air Force and trained – eventually becoming an electronics engineer. "The birth of my daughter sobered me up. Here was a little creature I could totally love. Somehow she softened my heart. I knew I had to stop drinking for her and I did."

In 1963 the slug he picked up in Korea that was lodged near his heart was finally removed surgically at a VA hospital. Several years ago, after his children were raised, he sought treatment from our psychiatric program. "As I was raising my family it began to bother me even more to think about the men I killed and what happened in Korea. I had gone 30 years without decent sleep and I needed some relief."

Walt was in the 34th Infantry Division in Italy. "I had good night vision and volunteered for every patrol I could. It was just how I felt. I wanted to get the war over, and I knew we needed to fight to end it." He became very close with five other men in his headquarters group because they always went on patrols together. His closest friend was a Mexican-American. They often spoke Spanish together, as Walt had learned it well while living in Guatemala and Spain before the war. Just before Christmas of 1944, one of their patrols was ambushed. All were killed except for one scout, including the five men Walt loved most:

> I missed that patrol because I had just gone on one the night before. I spent Christmas Day packing up their belongings. I was broken-hearted. A few months later, on my last patrol, I stepped on a mine in the dark. It blew my right foot off, as well as part of my left hand, and shattered the tibia and fibula of my left leg. Our medic stopped the bleeding with a tourniquet and gave me some morphine. I was moaning in pain with Germans closing in on us in the dark when one of the men hissed, "Shut up! Do you want to get us all killed?"

It brought me to my senses enough that I was able to remain silent despite the pain, and we avoided the Germans. Four men from our patrol managed to carry me to safety. I eventually lost my left leg at the knee, as well as my right foot.

Later in life Walt was never able to enjoy Christmas with his family. "All I tend to think about around Christmas are the deaths of those men I loved and the things we experienced."

Years later Walt and his wife retired to a little place in the woods. He got angry about a government decision. "I lost my head, took all my medals, put them on a tree, and shot a hole in each one with my .306." His wife brought him down to see us after that. For him the emotional wounds of war were more troubling than the loss of his limbs:

> It is much easier to live without my leg than cope with the mental anguish from the war. Though I never have regretted serving my country, I hated war and drank too much to try to sleep and numb my pain for many years afterwards. I never could share with my children how I lost my leg. I just couldn't talk about it, so I made up stories about sharks and alligators when they asked me. Getting involved in group therapy opened my eyes to the many ways the war has troubled me over the years. I have been able to enjoy life so much more since then. I even explained to my family what really happened to me.

After two years of successful therapy, he was the one who gave me his pack shovel with "PTSD SURGICAL EXCAVATOR" painted on it.

Sam was a sailor in his late teens on the cruiser *Indianapolis* in the South Pacific. He participated in many naval battles and amphibious assaults. His ship survived numerous kamikaze attacks. In July 1945 they delivered the A-bombs that were later dropped on Hiroshima and Nagasaki to Tinian Island in the Marianas. They then sailed, unescorted, for the Philippines. In the middle of the Philippine Sea they were torpedoed and sunk. No one picked up or at least acted on their distress signal, and they were not discovered and rescued until five days later. They went without water and food the whole time. There was only room in the life rafts for a small portion of the men. They were subjected to constant shark attacks. The sailors the sharks missed suffered heat stroke and searing sunburns, and many died of dehydration. Most of the nearly 1000-man crew survived the torpedoing, but less than one third lived through the ordeal in the water. "Men would go crazy from thirst and drink seawater and die in an hour." Sam learned to beat off sharks by "hitting them right on the nose." One of the worst horrors was "having my best friend go crazy. He just became convinced we would never be rescued. I tried reasoning with him but he wouldn't believe me. He gave up and died next to me in the water just a few hours later."

Swede, who attended group sessions with Sam and served on the submarine tender *Sperry* throughout WWII, was stationed at Guam, where the *Indianapolis* survivors were first brought in for treatment. He helped build freshwater tubs, into which the survivors were put to cool and sooth their burns. Swede notes, "The *Indianapolis* survivors were the saddest scarecrows you could ever imagine. When we put them in the tubs their skin just floated off. You never saw anything like it." Despite this, Sam re-upped and later served in Korea. Forty-five years after these events, he started therapy. It took more than a year for him to begin talking about the *Indianapolis*. During that first year of treatment the memories were so raw that he would break into tears and be unable to go on after croaking out only a few words.

I could go on with many more cases of "ordinary" combat-related PTSD. The broad strokes are all similar, but the individual details and responses are unique. Although the worst of the symptoms die down with time, they can always be reactivated with sufficient reminders.

What also must be understood and appreciated are the deep feelings the men struggle with because of what they have experienced. They have killed, either directly one-on-one or as a team or unit. Even if they didn't actually pull the trigger, release the bombs, shoot the artillery, or fire the naval guns, they know they helped others do it. They have seen their closest comrades killed and maimed. Many will say, "The best, bravest, and most caring of us died there." They have survived unimaginable scenes of gore and horror. These scenes seem to be seared permanently into their memories. They wonder about why they are alive and others dear to them are dead. In deep private moments they wonder how they can ever be forgiven and how anyone could ever really understand. When the symptoms return, they wonder if they are losing their minds. They struggle to share what is tormenting them. Despite their symptoms, these men show the great ability of most ordinary humans to face life's stiffest tests and still prevail in the end.

The following poem sums up much of what I am trying to express in this chapter about the ordinary experience of war and its emotional cost to the common soldier who fights and survives. It was written by a survivor of the "Lost Battalion," an American infantry unit that spent days surrounded by the Germans in WWI, never giving up. Less than one-fifth of the men survived. Those who did survive spent the whole experience with their dead and dying comrades, unable to offer them any substantive help as they ran out of medical supplies, rations, and even water before being relieved. The poem reads all the way down the left column before going down the right.[4]

Thots – Rhymes of a Lost Battalion Doughboy by "Buck Private" McCollum

Oh! to get away from it all,
Those war-ridden thots, that come,
To blind forever those memories,
And the sound of the bullets' hum.

To live once more, as I did before,
In peace and quiet and rest;
To just forget for a little while,
That it took from my life the best.

At night, when all is quiet,
And I'm lying alone in bed,
There comes a vision of battlefields,
The fight, the maimed and the dead.

Will I ever forget that hell "Over
    There,"
And the tales the battlefields tell,
Of the price my "Buddies" paid with
    "their all,"
And the place in which they fell?

And there's my two best "Buddies"
I can see them plain as can be,
A layin' "Out There" crumpled heaps,
And seems like they're calling to me.

I can hear the big'uns screech and
    scream,
As they go flying o'er my head,
They seem to say, both night and day,
"Remember the dead – the dead."

And sometimes I think, as I sit alone,
Perhaps it might have been best,
If I too, had paid that great price,
And were out there now with the rest.

Oh! those war cursed thots,
That haunt me night and day;
Dear God, be merciful,
And take them forever away.

The saddest part is that my job would be much easier if what I had to deal with in treating these men was only what I have presented so far. This is the basic trauma and burden of war. Now we must go one level deeper and look at what one of my vets so aptly called "breaking the Geneva Convention of the soul." This creates the deepest hurt and heaviest burden for the ordinary soldier.

Notes

1   Mumola, Christopher J. "Veterans in Prison or Jail", Bureau of Justice Statistics, Special Report January 2000, NCJ 178888. p. 1. This data is for 1998 and showed no real

difference between combat exposed and non-combat vets. Both groups were incarcerated much less than non-veterans.

2   Rothberg, Joseph M., PhD; Paul T. Bartone, PhD; Harry C. Holloway, MD; David H. Marlowe, PhD, 'Life and Death in the US Army', *JAMA* 1990, 264:2241–4.

3   Leinbaugh, Harold and John Campbell, *The Men Of Company K.*

4   Kalani, Jackie, *Vet Center Voice*, Vol. 16, No. 4, pp. 1–2. The original poem was in a small soft cover book written by L.C. McCollum, *Rhymes of a Lost Battalion Doughboy*, distributed by Disabled Veterans of the World War, State Post of California, Los Angeles, California, 1921.

Chapter 4

The Burden of "Breaking the Geneva Convention of the Soul"

I find myself struggling to start this chapter. It is the darkest pit of therapy for the common soldier. It is where my vets least want to take me but most need my help. It is where I am least able to help them. All I can do initially when I go there with them is listen and hold their hands, if they want, praying silently that they can get through this. When I first started this work I couldn't go there with them. I was afraid. I eventually learned what I was afraid of: they never told me anything so awful that I could not imagine doing it myself.

I had been conducting my WWII combat vets group for about two years. We were beginning to talk about some very difficult things. I was developing nausea each day before our group sessions. It wasn't quite anxiety or fear, but a type of apprehension nonetheless. If I had not figured it out, I would have had to stop the work. It was too distressing for me.

I had the opportunity to consult with a wise, older analyst named Paul Dewald, a professor of psychiatry at St. Louis University. I told him what was happening in group and what I was feeling. He smiled and said, "They are just helping you feel what they are feeling. That is useful for you and them. You can learn from it and better understand what they are struggling with. But you don't have to keep those feelings. You can let them go." In some almost magical way this interpretation of my internal emotional struggle worked. I was able to keep feeling, but not be overwhelmed. I learned to mentally step back and process what I was feeling even as I was experiencing it. My attitude toward group eventually changed from a dreadful anticipation to a confidence that I could patiently listen and feel without being afraid of what I would find in myself as my vets shared their worst experiences.

What I found in myself was that I had the potential to do anything, including the worst that men can do; but that doesn't mean I will do it or I *am* that potential. What I *am* will depend on what I choose to do. It was shortly after this consult from Paul Dewald that Ed was able to say in group, "Aren't we all murderers?" Instead of running from that question and trying to reassure everyone in group, including myself, that it did not apply to us, and thus subtly and/or directly discount what Ed said and block the work they wanted to do, I was able to listen, process in what way it applied to me (the real potential to kill in the right circumstances), and let each man explore what it meant to him. In all my work with combat vets, this was the biggest hurdle. Once over that, I was able to go where they took me and be with them in the way they needed me to be. They needed me to listen without reacting with fear, horror or condemnation. They needed me to listen and learn enough to fully appreciate the context of their actions. I don't have the pain inside me that they are constantly feeling when they explore these events, but I can now understand enough to help them express what they are feeling and start the process of healing.

These common soldiers needed to take me into four areas of pain and horror that are worse than killing enemy soldiers. These include the following:

1   Seeing and committing acts resulting in civilian casualties. This occurs very commonly in any major conflict.
2   "Friendly fire" incidents. Killing one's own men. This also happens over and over and touches most combatants.
3   Killing while filled with hate, rage or something like elation. This is also common.
4   "Battlefield justice": Vigilante actions in the context of war. This includes both acting as a vigilante and permitting or condoning the actions of others who do so.

It is important to understand that "breaking the Geneva Convention of the soul" is not breaking the Geneva Convention. The Geneva Convention refers to those rules of conduct in war accepted by most countries to regulate the treatment of POWs and civilians in war zones. Rather, it is doing things – or in some cases not doing things – that good men often feel are like crimes, and in some cases, people might argue are crimes. I believe those who argue they are crimes have not understood the realities of what people face in warfare. These actions are the inevitable consequence of war, at least the wars of my living vets. No war can be fought without them. It is naïve to imagine otherwise. It is also painfully misguided to make moral judgments about these events without understanding their full context.

We have already seen that for most combatants the dehumanized enemy eventually becomes human again. The killing in war becomes the killing of men and not the killing of dangerous animals or demons. But they are still the enemy, and although horrible, and at times searing to the soul, killing them is justified by the sanctions of war. As George Patton said, "No bastard ever won a war by dying for his country. He won it by making the other poor bastard die for his country."[1] These other types of killing (civilians, friendly combatants, killing with hate and rage, "battlefield justice") are always there, but they are neither condoned nor sanctioned.

Civilian Casualties

If you fight in a total, modern war in Europe, the most densely populated continent in the world, you can't help but kill civilians. But this is not what the combatants signed up to do; and it is dreadful and unacceptable in the hearts of the men who do it. Ed killed a little Italian boy in a fight over a stone farmhouse in Italy. Even though it was completely unintentional, he did it, and he knew he had pulled the trigger that snuffed out this little life.

You cannot fight across France in the 1st or 30th Infantry Divisions, as several of my vets have done, and not experience the following scenario. You are in house-to-house combat with the Germans. There's a sniper or machine gun nest covering the street from the second floor of a large home. Several of your men give covering fire, trying to make the sniper or machine gunners keep low while you and one or two others rush the building, throwing a grenade through the door or window as you hug the wall. You rush in just after it explodes, reflexively shooting anyone who resists or moves on the first floor. You see stairs to the basement and hear a noise. You lob a grenade or two down there, and then you assault the Germans upstairs with grenades and rifle fire. When the second floor is secure, you check out the basement. You find no Germans, but a French woman and her two little daughters shredded by your grenades. Sometimes you kill civilians on the first floor and even on the second. Sometimes it is all Germans on every floor and the basement also. Sometimes there is no one there at all; the Germans have withdrawn to the next house as you press the attack.

It is part of a dirty job and you just keep going. You try not to think about it as you prepare to do it again. If you hesitate when you start to press the attack, the Germans kill you or yours with their grenades and guns. They will kill and wound some of you anyway because they are experienced combatants, just like you.

Another daily scenario is at longer range. You are taking fire from a village or town, or in Vietnam from a group of hooches. You return fire or call in artillery or air strikes. Or, you may just know or suspect the Germans or "gooks" are there, so you initiate fire. They don't fire back because they don't want to give away their positions. You start to move up. When you are close enough, they open up and really let you have it, driving you off and killing and wounding several men. Now you are really mad, so you call in the heavy artillery and napalm. The enemy bunkers up to survive the artillery and then slips away – dragging their dead and wounded with them – just after the artillery fire lifts and you are starting your second ground attack. You occupy the village. The only casualties you find are dead and wounded civilians, mostly women and children.

It is just part of liberating Europe or fighting in Asia. It is war. There is no other way to do it without suffering more casualties or perhaps losing the war.

After the war, how do you reconcile what you have done? One 30th Division infantryman said to me:

> When I first returned home I could hardly look at the women and children walking around. They reminded me of what we had seen and done in Europe. We had killed so many and destroyed so much while fighting the Germans. How could we explain it to ordinary folks at home?

The destruction of the World Trade Center in New York City on September 11, 2001 was very disturbing to many of my 8th Air Force vets. They were sober and sad as they said quietly, "We did that in Europe. We destroyed buildings like that and even cities. Who knows how many we killed?"

E.B. Sledge recounts one of his experiences in Okinawa in 1945 involving the death of a civilian. His unit was sweeping through open country after the main battle had ended searching for Japanese stragglers. In one small hut he found an elderly Okinawan woman with a gangrenous-appearing abdominal wound in considerable pain. Sledge guessed the wound would prove fatal. She indicated to Sledge that she wanted him to kill her. He refused and went to find a corpsman. As they returned to examine her, he and the corpsman heard the shot of an American rifle come from the hut. As a young Marine, attached to their company headquarters emerged from the hut, Sledge questioned him:

"Was there a Nip in that hut? I just checked it out."

"No," he said as we approached him, "just an old gook woman who wanted me to put her out of her misery; so I obliged her!"

The doc and I stared at each other, and then at the Marine. That quiet, neat, mild-mannered young man just wasn't the type to kill a civilian in cold blood.

When I saw the crumpled form under the faded blue kimono in the hut door, I blew up. "You dumb bastard! She tried to get me to shoot her, and I called Doc to come help her."

The executioner looked at me with a puzzled expression.

"You sonofabitch," I yelled. "If you want to shoot at somebody so damn bad, why don't you trade places with a BARman or a machine gunner and get outa that damn CP and shoot at Nips? They shoot back!"

He stammered apologies, and Doc cursed him.

I said, "We're supposed to kill Nips, not old women!"

The executioner's face flushed. An NCO came up and asked what happened. Doc and I told him. The NCO glared and said, "You dirty bastard."[2]

When I read this, I know one man had approached the edge of the abyss and then turned and walked away. Another, thinking a little less clearly, had tumbled in. The consequences for the second will be long and painful. Back home this event will haunt him night and day. In his mind it will be aggravated by the comments made at the time by his comrades in arms. Many of our normal inhibitions are worn down in war. It is not until we try to reassume the standards and values of civilian life that the full impact of some of our wartime deeds bears down on us. Then they can be spiritually devastating. If an old woman was painfully dying of a gangrenous wound, was it so bad to put her out of her misery, especially when killing and death of the most gruesome sort had become part of daily life? What might seem almost normal in the hell of war can seem very different late at night, back in the quiet of civilization.

One of my patients, Jerry, drove a tank with the 1st Marine Division at Okinawa. He was doing guard duty at night. There were constant attempts at infiltration and regular night attacks by the Japanese. Orders and reasonable military practice required that if he heard noise and challenged and did not immediately get the password back, he should fire. Often if there were no Marine patrols out, the sentries fired without challenging in order to give the enemy no opportunity to locate them and shoot first. This night Jerry and several other guards challenged and got no response but the sound of running feet, so they fired. What they found in the morning were several Okinawans who had been trying to flee the battlefield. A little girl was crying as she held her dead father's hand. As bad as it was to kill a "dirty Jap bastard," it was so much worse to kill Okinawan civilians, and so awful to have killed a girl's father in her presence. Yet this is not Jerry's most troubling memory:

> Every time I dream, I see a young Okinawan woman and her baby lying in a ditch next to the road. She had her arms around the baby and they had both been killed by machine gun fire, probably from our planes. I thought at the time, "How in the hell could these two be the enemy?" After more than 50 years, I don't think I'll ever get that image out of my mind.

Can you put yourself in the place of these teenagers then and now? By 1944–45, most of the combat infantrymen and Marines were teenagers. Most of the WWII, Korean, and Vietnam War vets I have treated intensively were teenagers or in their early 20s in combat. How do they cope with the memory of these inevitable killings when they return home? It does not help to try simply to forget, nor is it helpful to share gruesome details with those who respond with horror or distress.

Sometimes modern warfare produces results that are more than even a hardened professional can bear. Manny was an airman with a photo-reconnaissance and bombing group that flew the navy version of B-24s out of the Marianas, Okinawa and Iwo Jima. He was in our WWII combat vets group for several years before he was able to share his full story. The terrorist destruction of the World Trade Center prompted him to speak more than he usually did:

> We were hard men. I had become a hard man at an early age because of all this. I hated the Japs and wanted to kill them all. It had been constant war for me: bombing, killing, living in primitive conditions with long, dangerous missions. I had seen awful things. I was no longer civilized.
>
> It was July of '45 and we had started a series of constant photo missions over a town called Hiroshima. Our squadron flew over, taking pictures every day for most of a month. I went on many of those missions. These were always rush jobs and top secret and what we developed went right to Washington. The morning of August 6th we were there again. On the way out we saw the Enola Gay flying in, but we didn't know what it was about at the time. We gave them the weather report that it was clear over Hiro. Then we didn't fly for three days. They didn't want us exposed to the air over Hiro.
>
> They then sent us back, 72 hours after the bomb, to take a close look. Back and forth we flew, slow and low, taking pictures at between 4000 and 8000 feet with our big cameras. At that altitude I could see clearly the horror with my own eyes. For two miles from the center there was nothing – no buildings, no

trees, no life. A few steel girders were all there was. The rest was dust and ash. Stone monuments you could see before, standing above a man's head, now showed up as little nubbins in the photos yea high [showing about an inch with his fingers]. Then after the two miles there were people crawling and dragging things and other people, but all burnt: women, children, everybody. You never saw anything like it. You couldn't believe it. You could hardly believe what you saw and what the photos showed.[3,4]

When we went home after the war we flew into San Diego. When I walked into the streets I was still like a wild man in my jungle fatigues with my .45 and knife. I saw women and children. They had no idea what we had done and seen. I started to cry, thinking about the women and children [and there are tears in his eyes and ours as he talks]. And then I don't remember what happened after that. They tried to put me in a hospital but I wouldn't have it. I couldn't go back and see my family. Not in that condition. I was no good for school or work yet either. I knew a couple before the war from school. I went to see them. He had been killed in the war. They had a five-acre yard and an old garage. She let me stay in the garage and I tended and cared for her yard. I was holed up in that garage for a year trying to be able to function again.

In the beginning of my career when a vet brought up something like this, my response to Manny and his pain would have been something like, "Well, you didn't drop that bomb." This would have been part of my attempt to distance him and even me from the pain of these events. Although this statement was true, it didn't apply because he felt so much a part of the larger team that did drop the A-bomb. And of course his plane had dropped smaller bombs on Japan with the same qualitative if not quantitative effect. Or to the infantrymen who inadvertently killed civilians, I might have said, "You weren't trying to kill those civilians." Of course it was not their intent to kill civilians, but their deaths were the result of "intentional" actions, and they knew it. I tried to somehow make an excuse for what happened – "It was an accident of war" – as if intentionally throwing a grenade or dropping a bomb could be an accident. Or, as if purposely shooting at running noises at night was an accident. I did not want to really look at the idea with my patients that they had killed someone and it wasn't another enemy soldier. I did not want to put myself in their shoes and think about that French woman and her daughters shredded by the grenade my vet threw, or the Okinawan family bleeding from wounds and dying in terror at night, or the charred, stunned, slowly dying victims on the outer edges of Hiroshima.

Being a psychiatrist, I have had suicidal patients who killed themselves with medication I gave them, or killed themselves because I could not treat their illnesses fast enough or well enough. This gave me a little taste of what my vets were feeling. In the end though, to help them, I had to stop saying in various ways, "There, there, it's okay. Its just war and you really didn't mean to do it." Instead, I had to listen to their real pain and remorse, and not shy away from its full impact. I had to be fully available to explore all the depths and permutations these acts had for them, acknowledging to myself at the same time that in their circumstances I would most likely have done the same thing.

Friendly-Fire Incidents

Every year in towns across the USA teenagers are killed while horsing around with their friends and showing off with firearms. Think of 20 million young American males in WWII being given weapons of every sort: grenades, machine guns, mortars, artillery, mines, bombs, pistols and carbines. All the ammunition is live. All the weapons are loaded. It is dark, chaotic; explosions with smoke and deafening noise occur. Add the millions of young soldiers from Korea and Vietnam. How often do you think they have accidents and kill one another instead of the enemy? It happens in every unit.

E.B. Sledge recounts how one Marine killed one of his closest buddies as they teased each other with weapons they thought were empty. One weapon went off hitting the other man in the head and killing him instantly. One man is dead and the other faces life changing grief, guilt, and a court-martial.[5] George Wilson describes an incident where a young recruit in the 4th Infantry Division in Europe seriously wounds himself and 16 other men in his company as they gathered to warm themselves around a fire in a stone farmhouse after a patrol. The recruit had taken the safety pin from a grenade thinking he might have to use it. He had then put it back on his belt without replacing the pin. It fell off in the crowded room and exploded.[6]

Although the above incidents stemmed from thoughtless playfulness and carelessness, the most common "friendly fire' incidents involve troops being bombed from the air, artillery fire at the wrong co-ordinates, and units getting confused and firing on each other in the dark. Almost all my vets with extensive combat experience have been fired upon or have shot at someone else in these situations. One sailor I treated, who helped man a 3-inch AA (anti-aircraft) gun on the cruiser *Raleigh* at Pearl Harbor says, "The worst part of that day for me was not the Japanese attack but later, when three planes from our aircraft carriers flew over. I helped shoot them down, killing the pilots – mistaking them for Japanese."

Ray, a sea-going Marine who manned a 20mm AA gun on the aircraft carrier *Enterprise* in 1944–45, talks often with tears in his eyes about the constant killing of fellow sailors and Marines that occurred whenever the fleet was attacked by Japanese planes:

> All hell would break loose as everyone tried to shoot 'em down. You know all those shells would go somewhere, and a lot of them came down on our own ships and killed a lot of our own men, including one of my best friends. The worst fear I had was being killed or killing other sailors or Marines by our own fire. It didn't bother me near as much to think about the Japs killing me or me killing them. That was what was supposed to happen. But for Americans to kill each other – that was a stupid waste. I don't call it friendly fire. I call it stupid fire.

This killing of our own leaves an emotional wound that is harder to reconcile with our deeply held values than killing the enemy. It can even be initially more painful than killing civilians because the soldier cares so much for those he kills. They can be respected fellow soldiers or close friends. Even if they are in a different unit or service they are on the same team. Still, they signed on for the war and in that way can be viewed as less innocent than a child. All in all, it is very complicated and individual, and so common that most WWII, Korean or Vietnam combatants who spent substantial time in the war zone have had to face either friendly fire incidents, the killing of civilians, or both.

Killing while Filled with Hate, Rage, or Elation

Why should killing the enemy when filled with rage, hate or elation be a special problem? After all, it is the enemy and not a civilian or a comrade; and killing the enemy is fully sanctioned as part of the intent of war. The following cases explore this to a fuller degree.

In Vietnam the Marine Corps created small teams that went out into the bush and villages and set up camp, often staying for weeks. They did not establish fire bases with heavily defended perimeters, but tried to beat the Vietcong at their own game by being light and mobile. Often they and the Vietcong would eye each other in the daytime as the VC worked his rice paddy as an innocent-appearing civilian, and then they stalked each other in twos and threes in the dark – setting up ambushes and booby traps.

Boyd was one of these Marines. His team was good and made themselves feared by the Vietcong:

> We ambushed a small unit. The next day one of the bodies was still there. We put it in various poses and took our photos with the corpse as if it was a hunting trophy. We mutilated the body in various ways we knew would be distressing to the VC. We set it out like a scarecrow to show how tough we were and to put fear in our enemies, letting them know what we would do to them if we caught them. It was part of the psychological warfare we used to make the Vietcong fear us.

Twenty years later, when I first saw him, Boyd was still troubled by this desecration of an enemy soldier. He knew this soldier "had a mother and father who loved him and didn't even know where he was buried or what had become of him." It was painful for Boyd to think of the joking and macabre way they had dealt with the body. "How could I do that to a man who was just fighting for his beliefs like I was?"

Drew was a paratrooper and a scrappy one. He was an outstanding boxer who represented his division in his weight class all over Britain and usually won. He trained other men in hand-to-hand combat. In September 1944, his division parachuted behind enemy lines to capture a series of bridges. The plan was to help British General Montgomery push a corridor through to the Rhine, cross the river into Germany's industrial heartland, and end the war by Christmas. It didn't work, although Drew did his part to the fullest.

In the airdrop he broke his foot and severely sprained his ankle, but despite that he gathered a group of men and proceeded to one of the bridges they needed to capture. They got there at nightfall. In the dark Drew led the attack on the guards. He crawled quietly up an embankment despite his broken foot and surprised one guard, killing him quickly and silently with his men watching from below, using the same type of hand-to-hand technique he had taught others. He felt a surge of elation as he killed the German and they went on to capture the bridge.

The broken foot became too painful and swollen for Drew to continue in the combat zone. When the British finally linked up, he was evacuated to England for surgery and a slow rehabilitation, never to return to the war. Back in England in a clean, civilized hospital bed, he couldn't stop thinking of the German guard he had killed. He wondered how any decent human could rejoice over killing another with his bare hands, especially when that other was no more than some young teenager "wearing a uniform he barely filled." Later, every time he looked at his teenage sons, he thought of his "elation" over killing a boy soldier. He was having the same trouble with his grandsons when he finally came to see me. He explained:

> I'm not sure I should even be here, and I don't know how you could possibly help. It is so hard to talk about, and I have never told anyone in my family, but this has been crushing me since the war. I don't know what prompted me to come. I guess I am at the end of my rope.

It is unacceptable for most of us to feel elation over killing someone. If we have to kill, it should be done with sadness, or so we imagine before we ever do it. Drew felt that he must be morally defective to have responded with elation to taking another life and he was unable to find any peace of mind because of this.

Killing with furious hate and rage often spawns the same type of moral anguish. Sometimes the enemy soldier is not just killed, but then stabbed repeatedly and cut up. His testicles may be cut off and put in his mouth just as you have seen the enemy do to your dead. You may be in such a rage that you kill the enemy even as they are trying to surrender. You may smash their face beyond recognition. Often the rage is sparked by what is seen as a treacherous act: a wounded enemy soldier might shoot your buddy as he tries to help the enemy; or pretending to surrender, the enemy might kill some of your exposed men as they move forward to accept the false surrender. Or, the rage can occur just because the fighting is horrible and gruesome.

A surprise or unexpectedly fierce attack can also generate killings of rage. When the soldier looks back at what he did and how he felt, he starts saying things to himself like, "What type of human could do something like that? What kind of a monster am I deep inside?' The memory of the event is difficult if not impossible to suppress. The memory of enraged killing often spawns a very negative self-message and the cycle of self-blame can be endless unless help is sought or redemption found.

E.B. Sledge tells the story of a surprise attack initiated by two Japanese officers as a way to commit an honorable suicide. The incident occurred on Okinawa after the main Japanese resistance had collapsed and the fighting appeared to be over. The two Japanese wounded several Marines with grenades and their sabers before they were killed. Hearing the firing Sledge and a corpsman rushed to the scene. They found one dazed Marine standing over one of the Japanese officers continuing to smash the officer's head into "a mass of crushed skull, brains, and bloody pulp" with the butt of his rifle. He describes the Marine as being "in a complete state of shock" with "brains and blood ... spattered all over the Marine's rifle, boondockers, and canvas leggings ..." His buddies finally took his rifle away and gently led him to an aid station. Sledge concludes his description of the incident with these words:

> Replete with violence, shock, blood and gore, and suffering, this was the type of incident that should be witnessed by anyone who has any delusions about the glory of war. It was as savage and as brutal as though the enemy and we were primitive barbarians rather than civilized men.[7]

I worry most about the dazed Marine who so thoroughly pulverized the officer's head with his rifle butt. Back home when he recalled his killing of this officer, did he ask the question I have heard many times? "How could a decent human being have done something like that?" Did he ever find someone to share this experience with in a therapeutic setting? I explore with my patients in therapy some of the darkest recesses of the human psyche. We have to come to terms with the fact that, given sufficient provocation in war, we can all behave in ways that later seem indecent, ruthless and murderous.

Battlefield Justice

Battlefield justice is uncommon but extremely difficult to come to terms with when it occurs. Each case is unique and must be carefully explored, and the full context needs to be understood before trying to make any other therapeutic intervention beyond supportive listening.

Dave had met with me individually several times when he finally joined one of my therapy groups. He left home at age fourteen during the Great Depression and lived the life of a hobo until he was old enough to join the army, where there was consistent food, shelter and decent clothing. He was deployed to the Philippines before the war started. There he was attached to the Philippine-American Scouts who terrorized the Japanese at night during the Battle of Bataan. He learned to slip out with a piano wire and a knife and silently kill the enemy by garroting them or slitting their throats. He saw killing the enemy as a necessary evil and was only troubled one time when he killed a Japanese soldier who appeared to be praying.

Dave was wounded and was being treated in a field hospital when the Bataan surrender was ordered. He refused to obey and left the hospital for the nearby bush. He was recaptured in time to participate in the Death March of Bataan and spend three years as a POW in the Philippines and Japan.[8] As a POW marching out of Bataan, he watched helplessly as Japanese soldiers disemboweled a pregnant Filipina. He survived the "Hell Ships," that evacuated most American POWs to Japan in July/August 1944. Atrocious conditions on those ships resulted in the death of many POWs.[9,10] In Japan he did forced labor near the second city targeted for an A-bomb strike. That city was saved because a haze obscured the vision of the bombardier enough that the B-29 went to the secondary target of Nagasaki.[11]

When Dave came to see me, though, it was not because of any of these experiences. Eventually he brought an old, scarred samurai sword to group and told us what he had done with it. This was what had haunted him since the war. Before completing Dave's story, it is necessary to understand some basic historical facts about the war in the Pacific, including the particular events leading up to the war's gruesome final months. These facts provide the necessary context to understand why the Japanese treated American and other Allied POWs the way they did and why the war in the Pacific developed into a war without mercy and, for the Japanese, without surrender.

Surrender in the *Bushido* code that ruled the Japanese military was an unendurable thought and an unacceptable action. Committing suicide was the only honorable choice, if continued fighting was no longer possible. At Tarawa and Iwo Jima, thousands of Japanese troops fought nearly to the last man. The wounded were left armed so they could kill themselves and more of the enemy who found them.[12]

When Saipan was taken and the first groups of Japanese civilians were about to fall into American hands, many killed themselves instead. Sam, one of my vets who served on the cruiser *Indianapolis*, was there at the time. He describes, with choked words and tears in his eyes, the shock of watching: "as hundreds of women threw their children off a high cliff and then jumped in afterwards. Some of the dead women and children floated on the surface clear out to the ship." He notes that over the next few days, "the smell and the flies" added to the horror as their ship remained in that area.[13,14] At Okinawa over 100,000 Japanese troops defended the island. Most fought to the bitter end. When the island was secured in June 1945, less than 10,000 had surrendered, and most of these were Koreans.[15]

As a warm-up for the invasion of the Japanese home islands, the battle for Okinawa portended that those final invasions would be bloodbaths beyond comprehension. At least 185,000 troops and civilians died on both sides at Okinawa – many more than those killed by the atom bomb at Hiroshima.[16,17] American casualties included almost 13,000 killed and nearly 40,000 wounded, plus 26,000 additional battlefield psychiatric casualties.[18,19,20]

The Japanese had lost so many of their skilled pilots by 1945 that they were no longer able to fight effectively from the air by the traditional methods of bombing and strafing. They resorted to using their poorly trained pilots in kamikaze missions. Flying across 350 miles of open water from Kyushu to Okinawa through a gauntlet of defending fighter planes, only a small percentage of the kamikazes got through; but the pilot-guided flying bombs still destroyed more ships and killed and wounded twice as many American sailors as were killed and wounded at Pearl Harbor.[21] The Japanese were saving more than 5000 planes and pilots for when the Americans were closer and easier to destroy.[22] The Japanese Navy attempted suicide missions, but the distance and American air power thwarted them. Japan had thousands of *kaitans* and midget submarines to repel the final invasions. The *kaitans* were large torpedoes with mini periscopes; a prone seaman inside guided the torpedo to its target in the Japanese Navy's version of their air force's kamikaze or "Divine Wind" tactics. Their range of only thirty to forty miles limited their use, but they were ready for when the Americans came closer. Because of the limited number of appropriate landing sites on Kyushu and Honshu, the Japanese had correctly estimated where the Allies would land and made preparations to exact the highest toll from the invading forces.[23,24]

Knowing how dreadful this combat would be, the US had minted 370,000 Purple Hearts for the expected American dead and wounded in the invasions of Kyushu and Honshu. These medals have been enough for all the American combat wounded and killed through Korea, Vietnam and Desert Storm.[25,26]

One final gruesome surprise to the Allied invaders would have been the execution of over 100,000 Allied prisoners of war when the last invasions started. The Japanese POW camp commanders were under strict orders to kill all POWs if it looked like they might fall into Allied hands. Their orders read as follows:

Whether they are destroyed individually or in groups, or however it is done, with mass bombing or poisonous smoke, poisons, drowning, decapitation, or what, dispose of them as the situation dictates. In any case it is the aim not to allow the escape of a single one, to annihilate them all, and not to leave any traces.[27,28]

That these orders would have been executed is not doubted by any of the participants. Dave, like the other POWs, knew this was what was planned in case of invasion, because his guards had told him so.[29]

On at least three occasions, it did happen. The first occurred on Palawan, as American forces returned to the Philippines. About 150 American POWs were locked in large wooden bunkers, which were then doused with gasoline and set on fire. Anyone who escaped the inferno was gunned down.[30] In Fukuoka and Osaka, Japan, at least three groups of captured US airmen were gruesomely murdered as the war concluded.[31] After the A-bombs were dropped, the Soviet Union broke the secret non-aggression pact they had signed with the Japanese and attacked Manchuria and other Japanese territory in Asia to gain control of it for themselves. They were approaching a POW camp where the Japanese had carried out extensive biological and chemical warfare tests on their captives when the camp commander and guards carried out their orders and killed all their POWs.[32]

Seeing death as more honorable than surrender, many Japanese interpreted the US surrender at Bataan (after the Americans exhausted their ammunition and food) as the Americans accepting cowardly dishonor over a noble death. They saw guarding POWs as the lowest duty a warrior could be assigned. It was dishonorable for an officer to be given this task, and this engendered bitterness, often taken out on the POWs. POWs were starved, routinely beaten and often tortured. They were prevented from escaping by the policy of linking the POWs in groups of "brothers," all of whom would be executed if any escaped.[33] Thus any escaping American knew that even if he got away, at least a squad of his comrades would be executed. Survival statistics confirm the grave toll of being a POW in Asia. As miserable as it was to be a "guest" of the Nazis, only 1.2 per cent of their American POWs died. Of the Americans held by the Japanese, 40.5 per cent died in captivity.[34]

Proud warrior that he was, Dave did not take well to captivity. He learned enough Japanese to avoid some trouble. But by the time he got off his "hell ship" in Japan in August 1944, he had endured starvation, solitary confinement and torture because of his lack of groveling – treatment that would have killed most men. He had seen many of his fellow prisoners die at the hands of his captors. He burned with a deep hatred for some of his sadistic guards.

In Japan there were two men he began to detest beyond all others. He considered them responsible for many POW deaths. They were brutal and merciless. One of these men was an officer over the POWs who had been with them since the Philippines. The other was the boss in overall charge of the factory where the POWs worked as forced laborers. On one occasion, while still in the Philippines, Dave made the mistake of asking for water. The officer heard this request and came over and laughingly pissed all over Dave's meager rations. This was seen as a big joke by all the guards.

One day while on a work detail in Japan, Dave was eating a lunch of a few handfuls of rice and a leaf of cabbage. A Japanese girl walked up to him and gave him her food "because I must have looked so hungry and starved." The factory boss went into a rage, hit her with a rifle butt, and then stomped on her head, knocking out her eye.

In his first group session, Dave drew the Samurai sword from its scabbard, handed it to us so we could all examine it, and began to speak. After telling us of many of the events leading up to August 1945, he then recounted much of what these two Japanese had done to other POWs and himself. He continued:

> In mid August after the A-bombs were dropped – of course we knew nothing about them at the time – the Emperor gave a speech on the radio that seemed to be a surrender speech. Certainly the guards began acting completely different. They were lax and careless, and no longer beat or insulted us.[35] I saw my chance and took it. With the help of two other POWs who did not know what I intended, I took the guards' rifle. They only had one by then, and all of them used it, handing it off when they relieved each other. With it I arrested the officer and made him give me his sword. This one you see right now. I took him behind the barracks and handed the rifle to one of the other POWs. Then I began telling the officer what he was guilty of, and I hacked him to death with the sword. One of my buddies, realizing what I was going to do, tried to get me to stop; but I guess he could see it was hopeless unless he killed me. He ran to get help from the other POWs, but by the time they came back I had left the camp with sword in hand. No one tried to stop me. I think even the guards detested these two men. I headed the short distance to the factory, hoping to find the factory boss. There I chased him down until I caught and killed him. I never expected to survive the day, but nothing was ever done to me by the Japanese. Both men's blood are on this sword. I never got it off. I never tried. Their blood is on me too, and I don't know how I can face God. They deserved everything I did to them, but even though the cease-fire hadn't been signed the war was really over, and I had no right to do it. God forgive me, I pray, but I don't see how He can.

The men in group reached out with love that day, but at the time Dave could not receive it, and it was many years before he returned.

George was 71 and dying of metastatic cancer in 1984 when I met him. His wife had died eight months earlier from breast cancer. He had made his will, arranged his financial affairs and "hoped death would find him soon." He was a mining engineer and had only retired because of his and her illnesses. He was at our VA to die, and do so in what comfort we could provide. The Chief of Medicine at the time had asked me to see George. He was a strong man and lived three more months. During that time I visited him frequently and he told me his life story. As he became comfortable with me, he spoke mostly about events that had occurred 40 years earlier in the Philippines, on the island of Luzon, where he had fought from 1942 until mid-1945 as an officer and eventually commander of a Filipino-American guerilla unit.

The guerilla war in the Philippines was long and merciless. The Japanese had superficial control of the main cities and towns, where they operated mostly in the daytime. The guerillas controlled the countryside, and as my vet said, "especially the night." The Japanese routinely threatened, tortured and killed Filipinos to try to get information about the guerillas. They imprisoned and executed many they thought were co-operating with the enemy. On the other hand, the guerillas were never above killing Filipinos who they thought were collaborating with the Japanese. Although most of the Filipinos supported the guerillas, they often found themselves caught between the two sides.

When the war started in 1941, George was working as a mining engineer in northern Luzon. He accepted a commission in the US Army. As a demolitions expert who spoke some of the many Filipino languages, he was a valuable man. When the Japanese invaded Luzon, he blew up bridges and roads to delay their advance. When the bulk of the Filipino-American regular forces retreated to Bataan, he stayed in northern Luzon and began organizing a guerilla unit. He used the tactics he felt were necessary to keep his men alive. That often meant "judging and punishing traitors and collaborators." The usual punishment was execution.[36] In 1944 the Japanese made a concerted effort to eliminate his forces. After some nasty fighting that ended in the guerillas slipping away to fight again, the Japanese took control of a town in the middle of George's area. They herded the townspeople together and threatened them with death if they did not help the Japanese capture or kill the guerillas. Since many of their sons served with George and related units, there was no co-operation. Then the Japanese issued an ultimatum. If the townspeople did not co-operate, they would behead the mayor. If they still would not co-operate, the next day they would behead ten more, and the next day, 100 more.

George had informants in town, so he knew almost immediately of the plan. Unbeknownst to the Japanese, George held more than 100 Japanese prisoners that his unit had captured in various kidnappings and night operations. The Japanese executed the mayor as they had promised. The morning after the execution, they awoke to find ten beheaded Japanese in the town square, with a clear message from George that for every execution the Japanese committed, ten more Japanese would be beheaded. That day the Japanese left the area, never to return in force. George assured me he would have killed all his prisoners, if necessary. He defeated the Japanese on this occasion by being just as brutal and merciless as they were. Despite this, of all the men I have treated who participated in this type of "battlefield justice," George was the least troubled by it.

Unfortunately George was long dead before I realized there was something important to be learned from him. My notes do give some clues as to why he coped better with what he had done. He was older, over 30 at the time. He had experienced the horrors of war for many years and was an experienced officer in guerilla warfare and devoted to his men. Almost paradoxically, he had a deep faith in a loving God. I never learned how or when this faith developed, but he believed he would be reunited after death with his wife. He held no bitterness towards the Japanese. He accepted that they and some Filipinos might have had reason to hate him during the war. He believed that death would provide the chance for reconciliation with his former enemies, and this belief gave him some hope of peace, even if it came after his death.

In April 1945, the Dachau death camp was being liberated by the 42nd and 45th Infantry Divisions. One of my vets who has since died participated in that liberation. It hurt him so to talk about it that I never got his full story. To many of my vets the discovery of the death camps was like the discovery of the murdered pregnant woman and unborn child was to Ed, in the very first case I presented. If Ed had found the murderer, I don't think he could have delayed justice any more than Dave was able to when he had the chance to mete it out to certain of his Japanese captors. Some of the American liberators of Dachau were also unable to wait for the justice they thought the Nazi guards deserved.

On April 3, 1995, *US News & World Report* published the following account of the Dachau liberation, replete with pictures:[37]

> At Dachau in beautiful Bavaria, a handful of incensed Americans joined in the
> revenge killing directly. Elements of two divisions, the 45th and 42nd, arrived

almost simultaneously. On the perimeter, the GIs found 2,000 bodies in 40 open freight cars. A hideous, decomposing tangle, the dead had been evacuated from Buchenwald a month earlier and raked by machine-gun fire on the train, the survivors left to suffocate, starve or die of exposure. The liberators stared disbelievingly and retched. Many wept with fury.

Fanning out into the camp, they found an SS contingent still there, guarding 32,000 enfeebled prisoners. Although a white flag flew from the *jourhaus*, the guards in the tower opened fire. The Americans picked them off one by one, heaving their bodies into a moat. The headquarters area was as well manicured as a posh private school; roses bloomed outside officer's villas, and turtledoves flitted in and out of birdhouses. But the prisoner's enclosure offered a fresh array of ghastly sights, among them an inmate whose genitals were nailed to a post. Is this the gate of hell? In the chaos of the next few hours, SS troops were rounded up – some rousted from beds in the hospital. A few GIs appointed themselves avengers, grunting, "Gotta kill'em, gotta kill'em." They machine-gunned more than 100 captive Germans against a wall with hands raised. Prisoners then moved among the wounded, finishing them off with handguns. "Pistole! Pistole!" the Germans muttered, inviting a bullet to the brain. Sickened by it all, Hank Mills of the 45th Division told a buddy: "We came over to stop this bullshit, and here we've got somebody doing the same thing." Mills, 22, had not seen his mother in three years; all he could think of was how much he wanted to be with her.[38]

I still wonder if one of the reasons my deceased 45th Infantry Division vet was never able to discuss this liberation in detail was due to his participation in this particular episode of battlefield justice?

At the beginning of the Battle of the Bulge, 125 Americans were captured by the Germans and held under guard in an open field near Malmedy. An SS detachment drove up in half-tracks, cocked their machine guns and opened fire, killing the captives. A tithe of men escaped and spread the tale.[39] My patients have spoken of their medics being intentionally killed by Nazi fanatics during that battle. The Malmedy Massacre and other events led some American troops to respond in kind. To even the scales of justice in their own eyes, some killed Germans who tried to surrender.[40] None of my vets have admitted doing this, but they were deeply troubled by what they saw done and the conflicting feelings they have about it.

The intentional killing of medics, contrary to the Geneva Convention, was less common in Europe than in the Asian theatres of war. In the Pacific, as well as later in Korea and Vietnam, US medics were systematically targeted by their enemies. Medics learned to go unmarked and armed.[41] That did not change how men felt about their medics, though, or how they occasionally responded when medics were shot.

One combat surgeon, Brendan Phibbs, describes his response and the response of his fellow surgeon Zimmerman to the "murder" of one of their beloved field medics by a Nazi soldier. They are clear in their minds that if they had known what this Nazi had done before they treated and evacuated him, they would have executed him instead:

Incident of the battle: January 11, afternoon, the aid station.

Training tells; the SS trooper is a dedicated, consistent swine, even with his right hand blown off at the wrist. Has he had a shot? Snarl, contempt. Does he hurt? Does he need help? Snarl, grunt, glare. He'd spit in my eye if he wasn't supine. Fuck you, Herman, we mutter, and we ship him off, bandaged. Half an hour later Zimmerman and an aid man come in. Zimmerman screaming, carrying a Red Cross flag and a pistol. Where's the bastard with one hand? Zimmerman's going to stuff the Red Cross flag down his throat and strangle him, so help him God. Pico's dead is why, and that prick murdered him. Not combat, not an accident, murder. Pico, I breathe, not Pico, and they tell me yes and describe the killing.

The aid man was crouching in a ditch with Pico, a hundred feet from a wounded man who was lying in the snow, his belly all torn with machine-gun fire, crying ... like a little kid hurt, his hands all red from holding over the blood running out of his belly. He kept calling for someone to help him. Isn't anybody going to take care of me? he was saying, quite clearly, and then he'd cry.

Pico finally told the other aid man he couldn't stand it. The machine gun was still firing random long bursts, but Pico said it was worse listening to that guy than maybe getting shot and, anyway, it was bright sunlight on snow, and anyone could see the red crosses on his helmet. He grabbed a Red Cross flag and ran out across the snow waving it. There was no mistaking what he was doing. He was kneeling by the wounded man; he had just given him a shot and was putting on a dressing when the machine gun cut him in two. The German was clearly having a lot of fun because he kept on firing long bursts into the wounded man and into Pico, keeping the bodies jumping and spreading red all over the snow. He'd used the wounded man for bait, an old SS trick.

All the time one of our patrols had been crawling up a gully, and they threw in a grenade; the German tried to throw it back but it went off in his hand ...[42]

The patrol that captured the German with his hand blown off appeared unaware of what he had done to Pico or they might well have killed the German on the spot instead of bringing him for treatment. Dr. Phibbs had treated and evacuated him before Zimmerman appeared with the full story of Pico's death.

Phibbs and the other combat surgeon Zimmerman begin discussing Pico's unfailing bravery in times of crisis and combat. They review together the many times he exposed himself and risked his life to save others. Finally Phibbs asks Zimmerman the following:

> "Would you really have killed that guy?
> Thought from Zimmerman, then, yes, he was quite sure he would.
> I wouldn't have stopped you either. War's war and murder's murder, and the more I see of war the more I know there's a difference ..."[43]

I often end up treating both the men who exact "battlefield justice" and the men who watch without preventing it. Avengers like Dave are often troubled. Some of the watchers feel just as guilty because they were unable or unwilling to stop it. Some of the watchers wonder why they were not "man enough" to mete out such richly deserved justice. Those usually eventually say, as one of my Korean War vets, Jed (see Chapter 3), recently confessed to me: "For the longest time I wish I had killed the bastard, but now I believe I would have been more troubled if I had and am grateful I shied away from it at the last minute." Curiously, he was talking about killing a fellow American whose actions were such that in my vet's opinion he deserved death for "cowardly treason." That cowardice had resulted in my vet and many others becoming POWs. When I start to see the scene through my vets' eyes and feel the pain and anger through their hearts, I wonder how anyone can condemn them. I only hope that they find solace and peace and that they remain open to therapy.

At this point I am mentally and emotionally exhausted from this discussion. I am sorry I have had to take you where we have gone. I am sad for the vets who have read this and had their own pain dredged up. I am sated on the horror of war and wish I could expunge it from the world. But we cannot. It is part of our existence. But to deal with it and manage it, we need to understand it. To understand it, we need to fearlessly face it and know that we are all capable of doing the killing presented here. War with all its horrors is going on right now in some form in one third of the countries of the world. And it is uglier than what I have presented. I have not spoken of the crimes of war. I rarely see men who have raped, tortured, murdered for gain or murdered to cover other crimes. They are few in my experience. They are deeply troubled and find therapy hard to embrace. When they have seen me, they have always fled in the end before they were able to get into deeper work. For several years of my career, I probably could not go where they needed me to go.

Some of those who commit atrocities of the worst sort do not have enough conscience to want to do healing work. Others are so convinced of their basic "badness" that they have lost hope. Many abuse substances and die young. Their stories could be the focus of another book. In this book I am concentrating on the war burdens of the common soldier, including those common soldiers who feel they have "broken the Geneva Convention of the soul."

Notes

1   Reference Patton's opening speech as presented in the movie "Patton".
2   Sledge, E.B. op. cit. pp. 293–4.
3   Hiroshima was the headquarters of a Japanese army with a garrison of 25,000 men and the main port of departure for supplies and troops going to Kyushu – the first of the Japanese home islands that was scheduled for invasion on November 1, 1945. Allen op. cit. p. 270.
4   Hiroshima-Nagasaki Publishing Committee, *Hiroshima-Nagasaki*, Japan, 1978 p. 41. The older of these two boys pushed his cart with his little brother inside five to six kilometers from Nagasaki before they died of their burns and radiation exposure. Insert between pages 136–7 and p. 200. These are photos that give some idea of the destruction to Hiroshima from the A-bomb.
5   Sledge op. cit. pp. 319–20.
6   Wilson, George, *If You Survive*, pp. 216–19.
7   Sledge op. cit. pp. 316–17.
8   Fitzpatrick, Bernard T., *The Hike into the Sun*. This is an excellent firsthand account of the Death March and the life of a POW of the Japanese.
9   Ibid pp. 189–95.
10 Toland, John, *The Rising Sun*, pp. 676–81, 712–15. Provides more detail on the "Hell Ships."
11 Craig, William, *The Fall of Japan*, pp. 85–6.
12 Allen op. cit. pp. 154–71.
13 Toland op. cit. pp. 588–90.
14 Allen op. cit. p. 167.
15 Craig op. cit pp. 13–14.
16 Allen op. cit. p. 270.
17 Toland op. cit. p. 820. Toland puts the number killed at Okinawa at almost 200,000.
18 Craig op. cit. p. 16.
19 Sledge op. cit. pp. 321–2.
20 Polmar op. cit. pp. 55–6.
21 Allen op. cit. pp. 33, 110.
22 Craig op. cit. pp. 42–45.
23 Ibid pp. 42–45.

24   Allen op. cit. pp. 226–7, 236–7.
25   Polmar op. cit. pp. 55–6.
26   Allen op. cit. p. 272.
27   Sides, Hampton, *Ghost Soldiers*, p. 24.
28   Allen op. cit. pp. 284–5.
29   Fitzpatrick op. cit. p. 210.
30   Sides op. cit. pp. 12–17.
31   Craig op. cit. pp. 141–3, 214–15, 297.
32   Allen op. cit. pp. 284–5.
33   Fitzpatrick op. cit. p. 155.
34   Skelton, W. and N. Skelton, "Environmental Trauma in Former Prisoners of War", *Federal Practitioner*, May 1995, pp. 42–54.
35   Fitzpatrick op. cit. pp. 213–20.
36   Volckmann, R.W., *We Remained*, pp. 125–6. Describes similar activities in dealing with Filipino collaborators.
37   *U.S. News & World Report* April 3, 1995 pp. 50–65. Written by Gerald Parshall.
38   Ibid pp. 59–60.
39   Toland, John *Battle: The Story of the Bulge*, pp. 67–9, 71–2, 331.
40   Ibid pp. 331, 337–8.
41   Bradley, James, *Flags of our Fathers*, pp. 66, 139, 236.
42   Phibbs op. cit. pp. 135–6.
43   Ibid p. 137.

Chapter 5

The Rules of Fear

Before beginning our chapters on healing and recovery, I want to look deeper at what my vets have taught me about the role of fear and anxiety in the development and maintenance of war-related PTSD. Many in the general public, and even some therapists, have misconceptions about this. I present five rules about fear that can clarify and correct these misconceptions.

Two major problems – the burden of killing and the traumatic loss of their most beloved comrades – continue to trouble men much more over the course of their lives than do the traditional symptoms of PTSD, including those related to fear.

Rule One: Everyone is afraid, but the vast majority keeps fighting anyway

When I first started to work with combat vets, I thought fear or anxiety was the root of vets' problems. I assumed that the men who were having difficulties and needed treatment were simply overwhelmed by fear. I learned instead that most combatants have faced what to the uninitiated would be unimaginable levels of fear. In doing so they conquered their fear and their fear of fear. One Marine rifleman expressed this very clearly:

> I got used to fear. It was like a scar or a limp that I had to learn to live with. I learned always to control what showed in my face, my hands and my voice. And I let it rage on inside. I never lost my fear, but I lost my fear of fear, because it became such a familiar thing.[1]

Every experienced combatant to whom I show the above quote responds the same way: "That's just how it was." All were afraid. Almost all got used to fear and learned to function in spite of it. Fear became familiar and lost its ability to control them.

The three psychiatrists working with the 8th Air Force in 1942–43 describe the progression they noted in the combatants as they were initially exposed to air combat, faced and then controlled their fear, and became effective fighting men. They first make the point that all combatants experienced fear, "All airmen engaged in combat experienced fear and it was a subject that they talked of freely among themselves. There was no shame involved in admitting fear or being scared and to the airmen such an admission carried no implication of being 'yellow' or a coward ..."[2]

Speaking of the typical airman who had flown ten to 15 combat missions, they say: "... the man had experienced fear and by now knew that he could deal effectively with it ..." Again speaking of combatants in general who had flown this many missions, they add, "... they attained a sort of tranquility in spite of their anxiety."[3]

The psychiatrists saw this fear as completely normal and rational, given what the men faced. Speaking of the air combat situation in late 1942 and the first half of 1943, they noted, "The stress imposed on the combat crews was of a severe order during the greater part of this year. On a statistical basis the crews had little chance of survival and only a small proportion did survive ..."[4]

A small number of men either initially refused to get on the planes when they got to England or refused after going on one or two combat missions and seeing what they were really up against. During that first year of combat for the US Army Air Force in England, only 50 officers were sent to the central medical board of the 8th Air Force for assessment that would lead to treatment, reassignment, or court martial because they refused to fly or developed symptoms that had no biological basis other than fear.[5] Another 19 officers were dealt with at the local squadron or group level, and a total of 97 enlisted men were dealt with at all levels with similar presentations.[6] Thus, out of the thousands of airmen flying combat missions at this time for the US Army Air Force in England, only 166 refused to fly out of fear or cowardice. The psychiatrists on the scene described those who refused to fly as suffering from "psychological failure." They stated, "... These men let the instinct of self-preservation outweigh their sense of duty and by means of symptoms made a separate peace with the enemy."[7]

The numbers were so small that the doctors wondered at one point if they were missing men who used real wounds to avoid further combat. They asked the squadron medical officers, "Have you had any cases who suffered actual wounds or disease but in whom the symptoms lasted too long, that is, were used to avoid return to combat flying?" They summed up the replies in these words: "The average opinion seemed to be that of a squadron surgeon who stated: 'Just the opposite seems to be true. The men do not generally use real symptoms to evade flying. They all seem to want to get back as soon as possible.' "[8]

Unless you have done the type of work I have done for years or were on the scene of battle as these psychiatrists were, it may be hard to appreciate the meaning of that statement. Faced with almost certain death, the vast majority of thousands of ordinary men kept climbing into their planes and performing their missions. They did this until they were killed, became POWs or were wounded to such a degree they could not recover to return to combat.

As I mentioned in Chapter 2, the psychiatrists made a serious effort to predict who would break down and who wouldn't. They looked at both those who experienced "psychological failure" and those who finally broke down after numerous harrowing missions because of "operational fatigue." Since they had been unable to find any predictive factors for either type of breakdown (except facing combat flying in the case of "psychological failure"; and flying hard, long missions several days in a row for "operational fatigue"), they asked the squadron and group surgeons if they had seen anything predictive of eventual breakdown. They summed up the responses they received by noting, "... These medical officers frequently remarked that they were surprised by the men who did become psychiatric casualties and were equally surprised that certain individuals whom they had suspected would not stand up to combat, did so with apparent ease ..."[9]

What is clear both from their work and my clinical experience is that all combatants experience fear, but most continue to perform their duties effectively. Very few men refuse to fight, and few break down later due to fear. One of my patients, Fred, spent a year in Vietnam leading a helicopter assault company, or "lift company," as it was called. They often flew missions into direct enemy fire. They lost many pilots and crewmen, but in that year they had only one mission when a man in the unit refused to fly out of fear:

> We were all afraid, sometimes shaking and almost sick with fear, but all of us kept doing our job. The one who finally refused was a macho ex-cop. His refusal really surprised me. He was the only one in about a hundred pilots and co-pilots. None of the enlisted men ever backed out that I knew of.

Jed (see Chapter Three), who fought in some of Korea's worst battles in the winter of 1950–51, remembers that everyone was afraid, but most did their duty anyway. "Guys were so shook-up they couldn't talk, but they still did what they had to do. You develop a tremendous respect for a person like that."

Although most men will do their duty in combat despite facing what appears to be near certain death, almost every man I have discussed this with in detail will describe at least one episode in their combat experience where they feel fear briefly overwhelmed them. It might better be said that more than 90 per cent of the time, more than 90 per cent of men do their duty in combat despite their fear.

Men of all types of personalities and backgrounds have the ability to join together as a powerful team and successfully face the very worst war has to offer. The bonds of love and trust they make with each other overcome the fear that would result in their fleeing the battle and abandoning their comrades.

Rule Two: Fear does not cause men to break down nearly as often as broken hearts do

The most successful fighting teams have the deepest bonds of love and trust between the team members. These deep bonds cause the surviving combatants to pay a high price in grief when the other team members are killed. The abrupt and brutal traumatic losses in war all occur in a state of high arousal, making the losses all that more painful and memorable. My initial training in psychiatry did little to help me to recognize the primacy of traumatic grief as a cause of combatants' symptoms and misery.

While training as a psychiatric resident at Yale in the early 1980s and working at the West Haven VAMC, I was shown a documentary film entitled "Let There Be Light." This film was produced by John Huston, the famous Hollywood producer, for the US Army in the late spring of 1945 as WWII in Europe was ending. It was filmed at Mason General Hospital, a stateside US Army hospital that specialized in the care of neuropsychiatric casualties.

The film opens with the statement, "About 20 per cent of all battle casualties in the American Army during WWII were of a neuropsychiatric nature." It goes on to state, "No scenes were staged. The cameras merely recorded what took place ..." The film presents what the US Army psychiatrists at this hospital seemed to think about the causes of neuropsychiatric breakdown in combat. The narrator states of the veterans treated there, "These things they have in common: ... Unceasing fear and apprehension, a sense of impending disaster, a feeling of hopelessness and utter isolation." The whole thrust of the production is that in the end, men become psychiatric casualties because they are overwhelmed by their fear of death. This was the message I was given in my residency training before I actually started treating veterans and my eyes were opened to a different reality.

Several years after I became chief of psychiatry at the Boise VAMC, George Smith came to see me. Because the Army nurse he married during WWII was from Idaho, he had moved to Idaho and lived here since shortly after the war. He was nearing the end of a successful career as a cameraman and producer of documentary films of all types. In the spring of 1945, when John Huston's lead cameraman became ill, George had stepped in and filmed most of the scenes of "Let There Be Light." He came to our VA looking for someone who might have some expertise in the area of combat neuroses. He was thinking about making an updated sequel to the film. Although he has not made the sequel, he provided me considerable insight into the making of the original film and helped me get a copy for my own use.

As I reviewed the film multiple times, several things I didn't notice or appreciate when I saw it as a psychiatric resident struck me. First, the cases presented were a mix of both combatants and men who had psychiatric problems but who never had any combat exposure. Second, it was clear from the snippets of actual therapy sessions shown that the psychiatrists themselves were starting from the premise that the men broke down from fear. Third, a careful analysis of what the men actually said and implied underscored that the most likely causes of their coming to medical attention were grief and depression, not fear. Since the film is difficult to obtain, I have transcribed below the entire dialogue of the longest snippets of all the therapy sessions involving actual combat vets. I will keep the psychiatrist's comments on the left of the page and the patient's comments to the right in chronological order. In parentheses are my efforts to describe some of the nonverbal action.

Case One

Psychiatrist   Patient
"And then after you got wounded what
happened?"

                                                  (very sad, lost expression and jittery)

"Same things only worse?"

"No ... seemed like my nerves keep getting worse all the time ... these airplanes, they bombed us. I got killed nearly by one."

"You nearly got killed. Where were you at the time?"

"St. Lo, I believe, somewhere ... don't quite remember ..."

"What were you doing when the planes came over?"

"I was in a hole ..."(Stares upward with a startled expression and appears to me to be having a flashback to the bombing)

"Do you know where you are?"

"I think I'm in the States now. They told me I was coming back. But they told me I was going to die. In the hospital I wouldn't eat hardly ... but I was sick. I wouldn't eat hardly. Told me ... I was going to die ... if I didn't eat. I told 'em I didn't care whether I died or not."

(speaking calmly and quietly) "We will see you don't die. You won't die."

(patient looks away) (end of snippet of session)

It is very likely the psychiatrist did not know at that time what happened at St. Lo. American planes almost assuredly bombed the patient and his unit. We had air superiority over Normandy; and there were few effective air raids carried out by the Germans. Then, even more than now, the military kept major "friendly fire" incidents quiet. At St. Lo, a 1000-plane, heavy bomber raid was staged to break a mile-wide hole in the German lines and help the Allies break out of the stalemate in the hedgerows of Normandy. Unfortunately the first bombs dropped short, devastating an American division, killing the general who was to lead the attack, and delaying the assault one day. The raid did make the breakout possible, as the front line German positions were also destroyed.[10]

Here we have a young infantryman who has already been wounded but has stayed with or has returned to his unit prior to the devastating bombing.

The bombing then probably destroys most of his outfit. The men he has grown to love are killed or wounded. He becomes so distraught by this that he stops eating. He suffers from anxiety and hyper-alertness, but he does not break down from this. The symptoms he describes and his expressions are much more those of overwhelming depression and grief, confirmed by the statement, "I told 'em I didn't care whether I died or not." That is not the statement of someone who has broken down due to fear of death, but instead from intolerable traumatic grief. As one of my vets said to me, "When my best friend was killed, my soul died." I believe this is what happened to this combatant.

Case Two

Psychiatrist

Patient
(calm but sad, with a Ranger patch on his shoulder) "Well I lost my last buddy up there, little Norman. He was 2nd scout and I was 1st scout. Things were all mixed up there. They were shelling us ..."

(interrupting) "Did that make you nervous?"

(ignoring the interruption and going on) "I should have been 1st scout. I was 1st scout and I should have been out in front. He was out and I started to go out after him and he got shot. And he said, 'Oh Dutch, I'm hit', and he crawled to my feet. And I started calling for the medic. I went back to see if I could get the medic and there wasn't any. I started to go out after him again and they wouldn't let me go. He was the last one of the original boys that were with me. Him and I were the last two left out of the original ..."

(interrupting) "And when you were shelled, how would that make you feel?"

'I don't know ... after Norman got hurt – er killed, why, I was all right when we were moving up or attacking, or anything like that. But when we got pinned down, I started thinking about him laying back there ..."

(interrupting) "And what happened to you when you'd think about him? How would you feel?"

"I just didn't care what happened to me."

"You mean you didn't want to go back into combat again?"

(speaking with intensity) "Yes sir, I wanted to go back. I wanted to stay there. I wanted to keep on for him and all them other guys: John, Striker, Tex, and Pop, and ..."

(interrupting) "And how do you feel right now?"

"I feel alright ..." (end of snippet of session)

This session is actually irritating to watch because the psychiatrist, who appears well intentioned, keeps trying to find fear as a cause for the soldier being evacuated for psychiatric reasons. He appears deaf to the deep grieving pain, and possibly guilt, the soldier feels for having allowed Norman to take his place briefly as "first scout." The soldier is a Ranger, the prototype of our current Special Forces, who has fought through the war to its end. In the process he has seen all his dearest comrades killed. He may have fear, but it has no control over him. He certainly does not look anxious in any way. This man has lost in combat all the men he loved most. Because of those losses, it appears he had one desire: to kill Germans in his dead comrades' memory without regard to his own safety. As he clearly states, "I just didn't care what happened to me." Probably an experienced officer, who cared for and valued him, could see this and ordered him to the rear – hoping to keep him from getting killed in some foolish action. Men in this state often care so little for their own lives that they will charge directly into death.

Case Three

Psychiatrist

"What happened?"

"Could you speak louder? I can hardly hear you."

"What was he, a Marine?"

"Now, I notice in this history here that you saw a vision of your brother. What a ... Tell me something about that, what happened?"

"Well describe the dream. What did you see in the dream?"

"All of you were home."

"You could see these images clearly?"

"What about this Mindanao thing you were telling me about?"

"You were scared?"

(interrupting) "What do you mean, 'If something happened?' Do you mean you were hoping you'd be wounded

Patient
(mildly edgy but very sad)

(speaking softly) "Well, when I was in combat in Mindanao ..."

"During the time I got worried that my brother ... He was killed at Guadalcanal."

"Yes."

"I guess it was a dream."

"I dreamt that I was home. My brother was there, and my other brother was home. We were all home."

"Sitting around the table, everybody was happy. We were laughing ... you know ... talking, just admiring each other. And then it ended there."

"Yeah, it was like in a dream, see."

"Well I ... in Mindanao after I got that amnesia, I admit I was scared."

"I don't know ... sometimes I hoped something would happen, then again, I'd say, 'Well if something did happen ...' "

and sent back? Is that what you
mean?"

    (firmly and clearly) "No."

"What do you mean by that?"

    "I meant that I hoped ... you know ...
I was just ... so disgusted and tired of
everything that ... I just didn't feel like
living. Then I would change my mind
and think back to my folks. It would
be a double blow if something
happened to me and ... I would be
standing guard, sitting on the machine
gun mount ... watching. I would hear
a little noise and I would let go ...
shoot. Wasn't nothing, probably just
an animal or something ..."

"Any noise made you excited and
you'd just shoot?"

    "At that time, yes." (end of snippet of
that session)

When I listen to this session, I long to whisper to the psychiatrist, "Ask
him why he was so 'disgusted and tired of everything' that he 'didn't feel
like living.' " I have some hypotheses. He was engaged in the Philippines.
American forces returned there in October 1944. The US Army units sent
to Mindanao in February 1945 had already been to New Guinea, Morotai
and Leyte. If he had been through several campaigns, which is very likely,
he must have lost many of his dearest comrades. One of my vets
experienced his deepest grief in the Philippines, a few days after losing the
three men he admired and loved most.

The vet in the film is implying that he hopes he might get killed. But
when he thinks about it, he shies away from that idea for fear of the
"double blow" it would be to his parents after the loss of his brother on
Guadalcanal. The dream of being home and united with his whole family
is just not possible with war's losses. There is sadness, grief and maybe
even depression here, but he did not end up at this neuropsychiatric hospital
because he was afraid of dying.

Case Four

Psychiatrist	Patient
"Do you feel worried about anything now?"	
	(very slow and quiet, with a twitch in his left eyelid) "I don't know."
"Are you mixed up?"	
	"Kinda."
"What's that pin on your shirt?"	
	(He raises his pocket flap to reveal his combat ribbons pinned underneath the flap so they can't be seen.) "My Heart and ..."
"Why do you cover those up? Aren't you proud of them?"	
	"Yes, Sir."
"You got a Purple Heart and campaign ribbons. Why do you cover them up? There must be some reason for you doing that?"	
	(He shrugs with a sad expression.)
"What happened over there?"	
	(He speaks slowly and with difficulty.) "We got in a scrape ... I was in a house there ... just got off guard duty. It was Friday the 13th ... sweating it out all day. A patrol came up – a German patrol. They shot a *Panzerfaust* through the wall ..." (trails off to silence)
"And what?"	
	"I was laying on a couch and right before it happened I got a little jittery so I laid down on the floor. When I got up again the couch was all torn up ..."
(interrupting and sounding very confident) "In other words you were almost killed? Is that it?"	
	"I ... Yeah, most of it went right over my head ..."

"Do you feel conscious, that is, are you aware of the fact that you are not the same boy you were when you went over? Do you feel changed?"

(with quiet sadness) "Yes."

"In what way?"

"I'm more jumpy ..." (looks away sadly)

"How about with people?"

"I used to always like to have fun. I used to always be going places. Now I do nothing no more."

(end of snippet of this session)

The soldier in this session is an experienced combatant. You know he is experienced because he had an intuition – some men would call it a spiritual nudging from God – to roll off a perfectly comfortable couch and lie on the floor. He immediately acted on this prompting or hunch. His life was saved, but what happened to the other men in the room?

The *panzerfaust* was the first rocket-propelled grenade. It was like our bazooka, but more powerful. When our troops captured *panzerfausts*, they kept them and used them against German tanks because they were more effective than our bazooka.[11] The *panzerfaust* could easily penetrate the wall of a home. On doing so, it would explode in a cone-like fashion, killing or wounding all the occupants in the room. The couch this man was lying on was probably right next to the wall where the *panzerfaust* penetrated. When he rolled off the couch, he put himself under the cone of the explosion, and that move saved his life.

Who else was in the room? When a company or platoon occupied a village or town, they would bivouac in a few of the better homes, where they would have some protection and be out of the weather. Seldom did a single soldier stay in a room. Foxhole mates, if not a whole squad, shared a room. These were the men this soldier loved most in the world. These were probably the men killed by the *panzerfaust*. This soldier escaped by following his hunch. Now how does he deal with this? Why didn't he warn his buddies? Why would God warn him and not the others? Did he miss the Germans sneaking up when he was on guard duty? Is that why his squad or closest comrades are now dead? These are the painful questions he asks himself over and over.

He is struggling with grief and guilt. He wears his medals, but they are upside down and hidden underneath his shirt pocket flap. He did not come to psychiatric attention because of fear. This was one of many close encounters with death for him. He was wounded and awarded a Purple Heart. Some time after this *panzerfaust* incident he broke down from grief and guilt, not fear of death.

Some therapists are prone to use the term "survivor guilt" in an effort to describe why some survivors struggle with issues of guilt. This term suggests that watching others die automatically leaves the survivors feeling guilty for having survived. I find this term very misleading and counter-therapeutic. Surviving combatants who feel guilty almost always feel guilty because they believe they failed to rescue or prevent the deaths of their comrades. These feelings may be irrational, because there was nothing realistic that they could have done to prevent the deaths, but they are based on more profound and complex reasons than simple survival. The vets need the opportunity to explore in depth the rational and the irrational basis for their guilt feelings. Saying those feelings are there "just because you survived" is a hollow therapeutic platitude that can leave important thoughts and feelings unexplored.

When I see the psychiatrists at work in the four clinical snippets from "Let There Be Light," I am reminded painfully of myself in the first few years after I began working with vets. I tried hard but often missed important points because I didn't know enough. I needed more training from my vets.

Shortly after obtaining my own copy of this film, I showed these interviews to my two therapy groups of WWII and Korean War vets. Their responses surprised me at the time, but added to my understanding. They were grossly offended that the psychiatrists seemed to be accusing these men of cowardice. They said things like, "What do those psychiatrists know of fear and courage? Did they ever look into the barrel of a German 88? Did they ever lay their life on the line for someone else? We were all afraid but we did what we had to do." My patients were also troubled by going back in time to 1945 through the medium of this film. They saw themselves in these young vets and it brought up painful memories. They summed up their critique of the filmed interviews this way: "That's just how our buddies and we looked and felt when we got home, and the response of those psychiatrists shows why we found it so hard to talk to anyone about what we went through."

Rule Three: Combat vets are not controlled by fear, but they are "hyper-alert" and have very fast battlefield reflexes, which are often out of place in civilian life

Because many combat vets appear more "jumpy," nervous and irritable when they get home from war, people make the assumption that they are afraid or anxious. They certainly have been afraid. They have faced fear of the worst sort. They learned to do their duty despite the fear of being grotesquely maimed or killed. They are definitely hyper-alert. They sweat at night and moan in their sleep as they dream of war. They get tense and edgy when they experience reminders of the war. They have intrusive thoughts of the war every day for many months, if not years. They hate it when people approach them from behind, but they are not afraid in the same way a civilian would be if threatened or shot at in a robbery.

They still have the conditioned reflexes, automatic responses and hyper-vigilance that helped keep them alive during combat. It takes time for these responses to wear off, and some of them never go away entirely; but they are not symptomatic because they fear death, even though they may appear anxious because of their conditioning. A small number of vets never seem to re-adapt to civilian life. It is as if once their nervous systems get put on ultra high alert, they just won't come back down. We try to help this group of men with medications, relaxation techniques, exposure therapy and a variety of other treatment modalities. They are conditioned to be hyper-alert, but they are not afraid. They just can't seem to get their nervous systems to reset to peacetime, and in some cases this can be disabling.

Rule Four: Combat vets remember being afraid and they know they should be dead, but they are more effective in actual danger than almost anyone else

A physical tenseness and greater alertness can be generated inside veterans when they think of the close scrapes and near brushes with death they experienced in war. They suffer through this physical response, which can be embarrassing. But most vets actually feel calmer in life-threatening crises than the rest of us. They are at home when facing threat and danger. The "adrenalin high" the danger provokes can even be experienced as exciting in a positive way. Some use the words, "Never have I felt so alive as when others were shooting at me and I at them." Because of this, many consciously and unconsciously seek out what others might term dangerous jobs. They become policemen and federal agents of various sorts. Many work as emergency medical technicians or firemen. Often they keep flying or work as smoke jumpers, fighting forest fires. I see them doing some of the civilian sector's most dangerous jobs. In comparison to what they went through in the service, these jobs are a cakewalk. Because they were effective soldiers, others see them as ideally suited for dangerous jobs and often recruit them for this type of work. A job as a policeman or fireman also promotes the same type of deep bonding with their comrades that they experienced in such a meaningful way in the military.

Ray, one of my WWII combat Marines, was leading a fire crew that was trapped by a forest fire twenty years after the war. The crew panicked and started to run. He yelled, "Stop! You might run from this fire, but I'll catch you and break your damn necks!" He was using his sergeant's combat command voice, and they stopped. They were more afraid of him than they were of the fire. Many young combatants initially feel the same way about their platoon sergeant. They are more afraid of him than the enemy! Because the men stopped, he was able to quickly organize them so that they survived the fire, which burned over and around them and would have killed them as they ran. They all eventually thanked him for saving their lives.

Fred, who had faced death many times from intense ground fire while flying insertion, support and rescue missions in Vietnam, spent a second career flying helicopters for the Forest Service. No wildfire was ever as frightening as combat, where men shot automatic weapons and rockets at him.

Often these veteran fire fighters, policemen, emergency personnel, pilots and test pilots are fine for years until one of their civilian comrades is killed. Then it seems that the grief they "stuffed" for decades nearly overwhelms them. "Bud" Anderson, a WWII triple ace, experienced this as a test pilot after the war, when a dear friend and fellow test pilot was killed flying a test mission usually done by "Bud" Anderson:

> In war, when there is death all around, a man can steel himself against it, block out the heartbreak, press on. But this wasn't wartime, and maybe I'd let down my guard. But of all the things that happened to me in my life, this probably hit me the hardest. I was a long time getting over it. John Davis was dead, and it could have been – probably should have been – me.[12]

It is a death like this, and the force of the ensuing grief response that often brings otherwise well adjusted ex-combatants into treatment later in life.

Rule Five: What vets fear most is breaking "the soldier's trust"

"Did I ever let my buddies down?" This question and its answer are what can trouble vets most. They fear letting their comrades down in combat and losing them more than they fear death. This fear swallows up their fear of death. One combat surgeon from WWII described it in these terms in his autobiography:

> In most of life love means coming to rely on someone else for detumescence or money or encouragement or company, but in battle, friendship (God forbid we should use the word love!) means readiness to be killed or mangled rather than fail the other men in a squad or a battalion; it is a fierceness of love and dedication unknown anywhere else, and a betrayal is a thousand times worse than the agony of a wife learning that a loved, trusted husband has just fornicated off with a secretary.[13]

I will explore many cases where this is a theme in subsequent chapters. For most combatants, no fear compares to this one. For many I treat, the worry that they may have somehow broken "the soldier's trust" is the "fear" we work on in therapy more than any other.

Notes

1   Davis op. cit p. 6.
2   Hastings op. cit. pp. 6–7.
3   Ibid pp. 22–3.
4   Ibid p. 4.
5   Ibid pp. 35–6.
6   Ibid pp. 35–6, 50–67.
7   Ibid p. 46.
8   Ibid p. 61.
9   Ibid p. 158.
10 Wilson op. cit. pp. 16–18.
11 Gavin, James M., *On to Berlin*, pp. 145, 205, 247, 311. Panzerfausts or faustpetrone were clearly a better anti-tank weapon than our bazooka.
12 Anderson, Col. Clarence E. "Bud", *To Fly and Fight*, pp. 252–3.
13 Phibbs op. cit. pp. 146–7.

Part II

What Vets Have Taught Me About Effective Treatment

Let me now take you where I wanted to go when we started this book but could not without touring hell. Let's begin the process of healing. In the next eight chapters I present the principles of effective therapy that I have learned from the practical experience of treating combat veterans for the last twenty years. In some cases they are standard therapies like group therapy where my experience with combat vets has helped me understand more clearly the unique approaches that make this treatment modality more effective and helpful for them. In other cases the vets have opened my eyes to therapeutic approaches that I had never considered, such as using reunions and "antidote experiences" in treatment. Though I talk about these principles in separate chapters, as a rule, many of these therapeutic forces are at work simultaneously.

Chapters 6 to 10 are presented in the order they tend to occur in therapy. In other words, the vet needs to begin telling his story first. Once he starts sharing the truth about his experiences, issues of grief and guilt surface. While this is happening, the process of education about PTSD and its effects on his life begins. As the work unfolds, the healing that comes from reunions and group therapy naturally follows. The use of humor and "antidote experiences" as therapeutic tools occurs throughout the course of treatment. Medications are wild cards, and as such can be used effectively almost any time in therapy when indicated. Most vets benefit from most of these therapies if they give treatment a fair chance.

Combatants are often left with deep burdens of guilt and traumatic grief. They have buried their feelings and memories in order to survive emotionally. Their sleep is disturbed constantly by grim nightmares, and their attention and thinking distracted by the intrusion of the grotesque images of war. All these things tend to drive them towards isolation and silence, or "bunkering up" as combatants often phrase it. Successful therapy involves sharing and honesty, mutual trust and support, understanding the past and limiting its power to control the present and shape the future. For many vets, choosing therapy means choosing to live a full life again despite the pain of the past.

Chapter 6

"It Helps to Tell the Story – But It's Hard"

No one needs to tell in detail what has happened to him and to feel fully heard more than a combat veteran. As they tell their stories, many voice something close to the title of this chapter. Creating a therapeutic relationship in which this sharing can occur is the biggest initial treatment challenge for the combatant and his therapist or listener. The vet must overcome several barriers in order to tell his story fully and benefit from the telling. The listener is challenged to do the listening in such a way that the recounting becomes therapeutic. The biggest barrier both face is the reluctance of the vet to talk. The material in the first five chapters gives some insight into the causes of this reluctance. I have found this reluctance to be based on three deep-rooted beliefs in the vets' minds.

First, I often hear something like, "Whenever I try to talk about it, I get so emotional I can't go on," or "I can't stand the pain of thinking or talking about it. I feel like I will lose my mind." This is a constant struggle early in therapy. The vet will say one word and then start weeping, unable to proceed. This even occurs when the vet knows the listener would understand his story if he could only share it. It just seems to hurt too much to talk about.

Mack was like this. He had served in the 15th Air Force flying out of Africa and southern Italy in B-24s on bombing raids over Italy, Germany, Austria and Romania. His psychiatrist was treating him with meds for sleeplessness and depression, but could not get him to process his war experiences, even though they clearly troubled him. Hoping that being with other WWII vets might enable him to begin working through his pain, he suggested Mack come to my group. The group included several other combat airmen, all of whom spoke about their missions and subsequent emotional struggles. Mack would try to speak, start to sob, get disgusted with himself and stop. After two years of gentle persuasion from other vets, he still had not been able to talk to us. He then left group saying, "I want to talk but I just can't, and I am not getting any better trying."

Herb joined this same group and was there part of the time with Mack. I had seen Herb on and off for years. He would take medication from me to help him sleep, but he would never talk to me in any detail about the war. I tried to persuade him many times to join one of my groups. He always said, "If I talk about it, it just gets worse and I have more nightmares." It is true that the pain often does get worse in the beginning before it starts to get better. I have learned to warn my vets about this. Finally Herb was having such bad nightmares during one stretch that I convinced him it could not get any worse. He agreed to try group therapy. I made him commit to come at least four times before quitting. He did, and admitted that although he still couldn't talk and the nightmares hadn't improved, he liked the guys and felt a little better knowing he was not alone in his struggle. Finally, after almost two years, he was able to start talking. Through tears he told us what troubled him most.

Herb was a gunner on a B-17 in the 8th Air Force. He was shot down over Paris in 1943 and spent the rest of the war as a POW. He describes that last mission:

> That last mission over Paris was hell. We were a close crew. I was senior gunner and manned one of the waist guns and was a trouble-shooter for the rest of the guys. We had the greatest little ball turret gunner. Every time I put him in the turret, Harry made me swear that if the plane started to go down, I would get him out before I bailed. Every mission I swore to him I would. We were getting shot up awful. The captain said it was time to bail. He would hold the ship as steady as he could, but we needed to go NOW. The other waist gunner had passed out from lack of oxygen. I got his oxygen mask back on and cinched up his chute, then cinched up mine. I could hear Harry's pounding as he screamed for me to winch him out of the turret. He had also heard the order to bail out. I was just reaching down to start ... I don't remember after that. When I came to I was in the air and pulled my cord. I had a scalp wound with blood streaming down my face. The plane must've broke up. Four of us survived, including the other waist gunner. I can't stand the thought of what happened to Harry. My nightmare is that he went down trapped, screaming for me in that turret. God forgive me! I never got him out!

Shortly after telling his story, Herb was diagnosed with advanced cancer. He hung on in group for two more years. Just before he died he came to group with his wife and told the vets that finally being able to talk through what had happened had brought him some peace. He thanked them all for listening and understanding.

The second major block to veterans' frank discussion of their war experiences involves feelings of guilt or abhorrence about things they have done. "If people knew what I had really done, they would never accept or forgive me. Even I can't forgive me." This fear keeps many from talking. It also bothered Herb, and so he never spoke of his shame although it haunted him every night. He felt that he would rather have seen his ball-turret gunner survive than himself. "How can you respect a man who gave his word, didn't keep it, and another died because of it?" Men make compacts like this all the time in war. They are sacred compacts between brothers, often made with all the fervor of their whole being.

Herb suffered with the nightmare of Harry's death for decades before finally finding the courage to come before a "jury" of his combat peers and be "tried." He saw the group experience as the "court-martial" he desperately feared and at the same time so much wanted to take place to resolve the question of his guilt once and for all. This "court-martial" concluded with these findings. The time between "Bailout!" from the captain and the breakup of the plane was no more than a few seconds. Because of his fast action one man was saved in that time – the waist gunner. He did not willingly flee the battle but was proceeding to do his duty when an enemy act made it impossible to honor his sacred covenant. The rest of the men in group always expressed in one way or another this thought: "We choose to throw no stones and see no grounds for condemnation." This "trial" in various ways was re-enacted several times with the same outcome. Each time Herb was a little more accepting of the "verdict."

If you have difficulty seeing why Herb's experience was so unbearable and nearly impossible to express, imagine that you are in this bomber in Herb's place and your beloved son is the ball turret gunner. The space is so confined that he cannot wear a parachute and cannot get out without your assistance. Every mission you help him squeeze into that little plastic bubble where, without armor, he fires twin .50 caliber machine guns, defending you and all the rest of the family from the attack of German fighters as they bore in on the vulnerable belly of the plane. All your beloved son asks of you is that if the plane starts to go down, you will get him out and hand him his parachute before you bail out. Every mission you solemnly promise you will do so, and all the family witnesses your covenant. But when the plane goes down, you don't come through, nor do you die with him. Would you have a hard time talking about it? What would you say when the surviving family members (crew) gather on the ground after the bailout and ask you about Harry?

Dave, who executed the sadistic Japanese officer and the factory boss in the "battlefield justice" episode related in Chapter 4, has never returned to group therapy for the "verdict." He has been "acquitted" many times since by his peers, as they have rehashed what he said and have discussed similar experiences of their own, but he has not been there to hear it. Some men simply fear condemnation so much for what they did or didn't do in war that telling their story in group or to an individual is like testifying in court before a hostile jury or judge. This can make it extremely difficult for them to start the therapeutic process, even though their listeners will never judge or condemn them in the way they imagine.

Some men "confess" privately to me after years of therapy but then wait many more years to tell the story in group. Norm was like that when he told the tale described in Chapter 3 of his "special mission." He finally told me in private, because he "wanted someone to know" before he died. He then made me promise that I would speak at his funeral and tell his family what he did and how it affected him over the course of his life. Since that time I patiently tried to persuade him to share his story with his family and our therapy group.

Norm had done the latter when he finally told his wife. She was temporarily caring for their grandchildren. Because of the crying children in his home, he was unable to sleep from nightmares. He spent the winter days freezing, puttering around in his unheated garage so if the grandchildren cried he would not hear and be forced to remember the little children he believes he killed. This painful response pattern had plagued him with his own children. His wife finally got an explanation for his lack of help with the grandbabies when he had the courage to share his story with her. She neither condemned nor rejected him.

I have seen one Vietnam vet for 14 years. He says our Chief of Medicine and I are "the best doctors a man could have." Despite that vote of confidence he will not talk to me about Southeast Asia. At first I worried he might be concealing some atrocity he had committed. With much more experience I know that is very unlikely, and that far and away the most likely cause of his muteness is the broken heart and shame he has about failing to save someone he loved more than himself. I know from his service record and the little I have gleaned from him that he participated in missions behind enemy lines. He was part of a unit that went to downed planes to recover survivors and bodies and remove or destroy sensitive equipment. At one point he tried to carry a man he loved through enemy fire to safety and didn't succeed. I know this because on one occasion he blurted out a few sentences about it before bolting from my office. If I say "Vietnam" or "Southeast Asia" to him, he starts to tremble. If I pursue it any more, he begins to weep bitterly, stands up and turns his back to me – often in the corner so I won't see his face. He chokingly warns me that he will leave if I go on. I apologize and stop. I dare not try more than once every couple of years. He struggles with severe depression, diabetes, high blood pressure and social isolation. How long do I have before he dies from the emotional pain that is slowly killing him?

A few weeks after writing the above paragraph, I asked my patient if he would like me to read it to him. He thought a moment and then nodded in agreement. Three sentences into the paragraph he was sobbing with his head in his hands. I stopped. He whispered, "Please finish." As I completed reading it he continued sobbing, but through his tears whispered again, "Could you please make a copy for me? I have never been able to share any of this with my sister and she deserves to know." He confirmed that what I had written was accurate. I printed out a copy and tried to hand it to him. He could not initially take it. Finally I folded it up, so the words were not visible, and placed it on the desk next to him. He gingerly picked it up and put it in his pocket. With his jaw clenched he got up; and repeating three times, "I can do this," he left the office.

The third major barrier to telling the full story is the veterans' belief that no one could really understand or tolerate hearing their stories. "No one wants to hear the whole story. It would take too long to tell. No one has that much time. And how could they understand anyway?" or "I have tried and it is just useless. You should have seen the look on their faces." There is some truth to this, and it has to be addressed. Often my combat veterans did try to talk a few times right after the war, with distressing results. Their listeners couldn't stand to hear it and asked them to stop. Or in some cases the listeners laughed and said they must be making it up. Sometimes they were told to "just forget about it," even by professionals. Sometimes the listener (the vet's girlfriend, mother, father or sibling) was sympathetic and willing to listen to the whole story. But the sensitive vet interpreted the look of dismay or disgust on the face of the listener at the grisly content of the story as a look of disapproval or condemnation directed at him, instead of the normal response of the uninitiated to the horror of war. He felt so condemned by this misinterpretation of the listener's nonverbal response that he stopped talking and wouldn't resume despite the urging of the sympathetic listener.

This happened often to me as a novice therapist. I had to learn to carefully school my nonverbal responses to the horror of war in order to help my patients tell their full stories. They feel so bad about some of what they are telling that they readily jump to the conclusion that others can't possibly accept them after hearing what they have done. They are prone to see signs of rejection in any unguarded word or expression.

War experiences are complex, hard to describe, and difficult to appreciate. Much of what is key to the story is basic to the combat soldier's understanding but completely beyond the listener's experience. The vet does not realize that others need to have almost every word explained. It is easy for the listener to get lost and confused. I am grateful to those patient vets who worked so hard to train me in the beginning! Their stories are hard to tell an internist in 15 minutes, or even a psychiatrist in 50. Before they dare to start, the vets need to know the therapist will be around and willing to listen for a long time.

Group therapy can be slow, and older arthritic men can't sit for more than an hour. Listening can also be tiring, and with all good intentions the listener can be worn out after a few hours. Many times I have come home from work emotionally exhausted and unable to listen to another soul. I am grateful for the restoration of a good night's sleep and an understanding family! It takes patience in both the teller and the listener to get the truth out. The story often has to be told many times, with new details and perspectives coming out each time. I have listened for years and am still learning new facets of what some of my patients went through.

Every combat autobiography and good war history I read helps me. These books give me the vocabulary and historical context my vets unconsciously expect me to know. It is surprising how helpful it is to know the basic history of divisions, battles and wars. It is helpful to know about weapons and training. The more knowledge and experience the listener gets in these areas, the more he or she can facilitate with understanding comments, rather than obstruct the process with confused looks or questions which are readily interpreted by these sensitive men as criticism or disbelief. What these men need, in order to really tell the full story, is hard to supply. I am grateful that the taxpayers of America are willing to pay people like my staff to do it.

Being able to tell the full story of one's war experiences to a sympathetic, effective listener, even just once, can be remarkably healing for the combat vet. Years ago the Chief of Medicine at our hospital persuaded a very reluctant veteran to come and see me. When he came into my office with his wife, he looked at me sternly. Wagging his finger, he laid down the law: "I know you are one of those doctors who try to get vets to talk. I've heard of you and I am not talking!" By his choice, since retirement, he lived an isolated existence with his wife in a cabin in the Idaho woods. His wife provided most of the history, although she knew little more than that he had been an artillery officer in Europe in WWII. His service record listed awards for heroism, a Purple Heart, and a small disability for "war neurosis," one of the WWII US Army's formal psychiatric terms for "battle fatigue," or what we now call PTSD. Even in his sixties he was tall and strong, but very tense and guarded when I saw him. It appeared that he had severe anxiety and panic disorder, with panic attacks occurring almost daily. Panic disorder is more common in men with PTSD. At the time I was able to get him off caffeine and on an anti-depressant. Those two interventions decreased the anxiety and the panic attacks stopped. Because of this help he continued to see me, but always with his wife. He never would talk further about the war. Finally he forbade me to even ask about it, or he would stop seeing me.

A month after Desert Storm ended he came for a previously scheduled appointment. I expected to see him much worse than usual because the media coverage of the war had exacerbated the war-related symptoms of most of my patients. When he walked in I was surprised to see him smiling and joking for the first time. He and his wife confirmed that he was much improved. When I asked him why he thought he was doing so much better, he was close-lipped as usual, saying only, "My wife can tell you." She proceeded to tell me what had happened from her perspective:

> When the air war started I really began to worry about him. I would have called you but he wouldn't let me. He was up late watching the war news – way too much of it. He was screaming in his sleep and I could hardly stay safely in bed at night, as he would lash out from time-to-time while dreaming. Then I thought he would lose his mind when the ground fighting and artillery started. He couldn't seem to stand to watch, nor would he let me turn it off. He could not sleep. He would pace back and forth in front of the TV, muttering and clenching his fists and at times giving out a yell. Abruptly he just started talking to me almost as fast as he could. He told me all about the war. He told me about towns in France they destroyed with their artillery and Germans they had killed and Frenchmen too. He spoke in great detail. He was with Patten's 3rd Army as they fought across Europe. He talked about winter combat. He spoke of holding one of his men in his arms as he died and weeping, and then he started to weep again. He wept as he spoke. He sobbed. He cursed. He spoke all day, it seemed, or at least several hours. I was exhausted when he finished. I wept along with him. I only understood part of it. When he finished he slept like a baby for almost fifteen hours. When he got up he said he felt the best he had in years, so I didn't call you after all. He has been doing great ever since. But he does not want to talk about it any more.

"That's right," he confirmed. "Once was enough." And he never would talk to me about it, but he died a lot more at ease a few years later.

The psychiatric term for this is catharsis. Some call it abreaction. A cathartic session means telling the whole traumatic story with all its meaning, feeling the emotions appropriate to the story as you do so, and having it all be at least somewhat healing. At times, as in this case, it can be dramatically therapeutic all by itself.[1] Usually we only talk like this to people we trust, although occasionally it can happen with a perfect stranger (like a medical student), as it is sometimes easier to "confess" to someone we don't know or won't see again. A cathartic telling of the traumatic story can be the beginning of real progress in therapy. The telling unleashes and makes conscious powerful feelings and beliefs that desperately need to be expressed and explored.

The story usually needs to be told many times and approached from various angles to get the full benefit of the understanding and emotional release that comes from good cathartic work. In most cases this is hard, slow work for the men and their therapists. We explore this process again in Chapter 10 on group therapy. Now let's examine an important aspect of war trauma therapy that we have touched on already, the importance of grief therapy.

Note

1   Grinker op. cit. pp. 7–9 and 97–102. This case shows the positive and dramatic effect of sodium pentathol-induced abreaction, pp. 18–19. This is another instructive case of severe loss and trauma with a positive resolution through abreaction. This book has many similar cases.

Chapter 7

Grief and Grieving

As I have previously noted, the two types of war experiences that trouble men the most over the course of their post-war lives are the killing they were involved in and the profound traumatic grief they have to bear as the "blood brothers" in their units become casualties of war. Fighting effectively as a unit demands deep devotion and trust among the team members. The bonds men share are fiercely forged by intense personal need. The good combat team seems welded together as if it was one organism. The nearness of death and the vital energy of fear and ultimate arousal make these war relationships at least as strong and interdependent as those of the best marriages. At the same time the beloved partner can be savagely destroyed in an instant. The survivors must brutally dismiss their grief and continue acting as combatants. They must continue to do their duty or have others die by their neglect or become casualties themselves. What is the ultimate impact of these brutal losses and suppression of grieving on their psyches and souls? This chapter is only a beginning of that exploration. It echoes over and over throughout the rest of this book.

Tim was a combat medic. To understand his story and the story of the other medics in this book, we need to look more closely at what a medic experiences. I have treated many medics over the years. Why should that be? They rarely kill the enemy. I have never known one who killed a civilian or who was involved in "battlefield justice." They usually are totally dedicated to saving others. So why do so many come and see us? Medics experience the pain of combat-induced traumatic grief as profoundly as any group of combatants.

A good medic is revered and loved by his men just as a good officer is, and for the same reasons. When they do their jobs well, they save lives. They also suffer, like officers sometimes do, from the curse of responsibility. They can feel responsible for all the soldiers they don't save. The combatants sometimes think their medics can save anyone. It is both a hope and a result of having seen their medic perform regular medical "miracles." The medics have the same wish. In most cases they have volunteered to be medics. They want to bind up wounds rather than fight.

Some are conscientious objectors and refuse to bear arms. A good officer loves and cares for his men. So does a good medic. Medics love enough to risk their bodies for others. They see the most horrible things, over and over: arteries, pumping blood everywhere, that must be grabbed and clamped; bones sticking grotesquely through flesh; intestines laid bare in filth; body parts missing or dangling by a skin flap; holes in heads with brains leaking out. And sometimes worse, their men pleading with them and crying, moaning in agony and choking on their own blood. All around them people are relying on them to do the impossible and save this one more horribly wounded man. Sometimes men are asking the medic to kill them and end their suffering, while their comrades are pleading for the wounded men's lives.

As they do their jobs, medics store up a lifetime of grotesque nightmares. Afterwards they play the events back and forth in their heads, thinking, "If I had just done that, he would be alive now," or, "Maybe I should have tried this instead?" So in the end the gnawing worm inside is still linked to killing, but in this case the death was of "the man I should have saved." There is also no escape from the pain, because wounded and dying patients are often beloved "family."

My patient Tim was a mid-western farm boy a long way from home when he landed with the 1st Infantry Division on Omaha Beach in Normandy, June 6, 1944. "For many years all I could remember about that day was that at the end I was covered in blood, like layers of lacquer. It had dried on my hands and glued my fingers firmly together." He served with the division as they fought across France into Germany, suffering 206 per cent casualties.[1] He put his body in harm's way constantly for these men and was awarded medals for bravery, including the Silver Star.

In late November 1944 Tim was sitting in a captured bunker just inside Germany. He started thinking about a man he had tried to save that day, one of the last original men in the company. He thought of several others he had lost or who were evacuated with terrible wounds. He began weeping for them, something he had never let himself do, but now could not stop. He sobbed rivers of tears. After two days he had a frozen beard of tears hanging to his waist. Finally his commander said, "Tim, you are a great medic, but you are no good to any of us like this," and ordered him evacuated. He became a psychiatric casualty and never returned to the front. He received little treatment and was repatriated and discharged in 1945. He tried to explain to his father what had happened but he gave up after his father misinterpreted what Tim said as his being sent home "for crying."

Tim did his best to forget about the war and get on with life. He pursued some education, married, and worked in finance and sales in New York City. Grotesque, intrusive thoughts and nightmares of the war continued to hound him:

> I started drinking to sleep. Then I drank to numb the pain. Then I just drank to drink. I lost my job. I lost my family. I ended up on the street. I finally got help in a drug and alcohol treatment program. I got sober. I started a new life as a drug and alcohol counselor. It suited me better, but I never dealt with the war. I remarried in 1974. Ten years later I was watching a special on D-Day. Walter Cronkite and Ronald Reagan were walking down Omaha Beach and stopped at a scarred old pillbox. I suddenly remembered that this pillbox had pinned us down and had been responsible for wounding and killing many of us! After we captured it, it became my aid station. The events of D-Day flooded back. Tears began streaming down my face. I started sobbing. It seemed like I could not stop again. My wife insisted I get help.

Tim finally got the treatment he needed. He needed to grieve in the deepest way. He needed to tell his story of pain and horror, of trying and failing to save men he loved, of sending them off dreadfully wounded and never knowing what became of them. He also needed to remember the ones he had saved as a balance to those who died. He was ready for this work, and he worked hard. He talked and grieved. He shared. He helped other vets do the same in several different treatment settings and groups. The intensity of the pain and grief eased. His well of grief became a fountain of compassion as he helped others explore their own pain.

This deep grief cannot be dealt with safely in war. The traumatic loss of men loved so deeply is too brutal, too much. As one WWII fighter ace so aptly said, "Grief could kill."[2] If a combatant started thinking about it, he could lose his edge as a soldier and become an easy victim of the enemy. That nearly unendurable pain has to be stuffed away. The good soldier hardens himself to these losses. One of my Vietnam vets put it this way: "When my best friend was killed my soul died. You have to just go numb after that to keep going on."

Sometimes, however, the loss is just too great to be suppressed. As we have seen, aircrews are very close. Imagine the scene described by this pilot as he returns to base from a savage daylight bombing raid over Berlin:

> As we circled the airfield alone we could see a lot of empty spaces. We landed and when we taxied to our space we found our squadron commander waiting for us. He was crying. We were stunned to learn that we were the only aircraft

of the squadron to return to the field and only one of four [they started with 20] to make it back to England. What do you say, what do you do when your squadron commander is crying and wants to know what has happened? You do the same.[3]

Audie Murphy, the US Army's most decorated combat infantryman in WWII, made a fascinating movie about himself entitled, "To Hell and Back." He is both the director and lead actor in this movie based on his autobiography. At one point at Anzio the replacements in his unit are complaining to the "old guys" that they aren't very friendly to the new guys. The "old guys" respond in effect, "We made the mistake of getting close to all the original guys and we won't do that again."

All combat vets are familiar with this emotional double-edged sword of war. They learn to love deeply the men with whom they serve. They must in order to become a good combat unit, but they pay the price of a broken heart as the combat goes on and the losses mount. To protect themselves, they try not to feel. They become numb if at all possible. One young platoon leader, after he began seeing his men killed in combat, described how he tried to protect himself from the pain of these losses:

> I knew then I'd never survive if I let myself get tied in with every case. It was vital for me to build some sort of protective shield within myself and concentrate only on what had to be done in the present and how to do it. I forced myself to suppress all thoughts of prior losses and gruesome mental pictures of the tragedy of war.[4]

Becoming numb, or building this type of protective shield, has a variety of consequences. One of my vets told about returning from Vietnam on leave to attend his father's funeral. He loved his dad but he could not let himself cry. He was disturbed by his own apparent lack of feeling. "What has happened to me? What have I become?" He did not perceive at the time that he was responding to his father's death just as he had learned to respond to the deaths of his dear comrades – with numbness. War allows for no other response if combatants are to continue to fight and survive.

Larry, a Special Forces officer, had prepared himself to lose some of his men: "No matter how good you are you will lose some eventually." But it was the loss of his young Vietnamese translator and advisor that hurt him most in combat. "I forgot to put up the wall I used with the other men." This numbness is the flip side of grief. Men end up exploring both at the same time in therapy. They often struggle to make deep emotional relationships after the war. The fear of suffering from profound emotional loss lingers on and haunts their personal lives. Exploring the grief behind the numbness helps both problems.

Most men hate to cry. We are socialized not to. It is embarrassing and makes us feel weak and foolish. I have a little lecture for new patients and new guys in group. "We cry here. It is OK. It is part of what we do. When we do it we know it is good for us. Don't fight it." The old hands smile and sometimes even laugh. They nod and add, "Yep, we have all cried here." Then, when someone starts crying, they often shed tears in support.

Although steeling themselves against grief keeps the combatants alive and functioning in battle, this learned response has negative consequences in civilian life. It is as if they have to suppress all their feelings to keep from breaking down. This habit of emotional suppression can become automatic. Normal emotional relationships with wives and children can be difficult. There is an unconscious tendency to get only so close and not fully open up the heart to avoid getting it broken again. All family members can suffer because of this distancing. It sometimes threatens vets' marriages. These wartime losses and the accompanying emotional suppression can also predispose combatants to depression later in life, unless they start working through these issues.

We have seen in the case of Tim how his pent-up grief was overwhelming both during the war and in 1984 watching a D-Day special. It was the same with JR. As I noted in Chapter 2, he began crying on the 41st anniversary of his last bombing mission, during his first year of retirement. He had walled off those memories so effectively that he cried for three months before making the connection to the grief engendered by that last mission. It has been over 17 years since his deep pain prodded me to start that first WWII combat vets group. Since then he has worked through his grief very effectively. Now I watch him in group as he softly and soothingly extends his love to help others do the same. Working through their grief and numbness can be a long and painful process for vets, but it is essential for them to feel fully alive and engage completely in the loving relationships of their current lives.

Notes

1   Ambrose, Stephen E., *Citizen Soldiers*, p. 280.
2   Anderson op. cit. p. 166.
3   Ethel, Jeffrey and Alfred Price, *Target Berlin*, p. 130.
4   Wilson op. cit. p. 22.

Chapter 8

Understanding Conditioned Responses

One important therapeutic process is the growing understanding men gain about the connection between what they currently think, feel, and do, and the war. They start to see consciously the connections between what they experienced in war and how it has been influencing their behavior and feelings as civilians. This awareness of the influence of their combat experiences on their current actions allows them to free themselves from the unconscious tyranny of their war conditioned behavior and assert firmer control of their present behavior – improving their current lives and adaptation.

Walt (Introduction and Chapter 3), who lost his leg in Italy to a mine, whose five dearest comrades were killed just before Christmas, and who gave me his pack shovel with PTSD SURGICAL EXCAVATOR painted on it, sent me the following letter:

Dear Dr. Dewey,

For approximately 2 years I have been attending your PTSD group therapy sessions along with other WWII veterans. As a result 2 striking impressions come to mind as I mentally review past discussions and shared experiences. Foremost, I have felt honored to have associated with the best, veterans who unselfishly placed their lives in contention but who unwittingly became casualties no less than those who sustained physical injuries. As a victim of both, I can state unequivocally that given a choice, I would opt for physical suffering over the mental anguish which ever lurks in the mirror of our thoughts. For whatever particular memories, which plague and gnaw at our conscious, the resulting damage remains as a silent partner to our pain.

Secondly, the veil of mystery has been lifted in my mind to reveal the reasons for many of my past feelings and actions. My mind has at last penetrated the tangled web of confusion, self-doubt, loss of self-esteem and guilt associated with my past. I still find it difficult to lay what I consider these failures on the doorstep of PTSD. At least I now understand even as I continue reliving the realities of war.

I realize there is no cure, no magic moment in time that will relieve me of my mental suffering. It is sufficient to know that to understand is perhaps to cope. So now I have arrived at that diverging road named hope. You reminded me once that the last whisper out of Pandora's chest was hope. Enter with doubt and exit with hope.

I will remain ever grateful for the help, understanding and empathy you and Pat Neeser have shown, and to my comrades who endured my outbursts of frustration and anger. The episode of the medals might be considered childish but to me was symbolic of the disgust I feel towards the insanity of war, and to those who placed a value on patriotism. So be it!

Again I thank each and everyone. I won't say good-by as I may have to return for a retread.

Walt uses several phrases that are the theme of this chapter: "The veil of mystery has been lifted," "My mind has at last penetrated the tangled web of confusion," "I now understand even as I continue reliving," "To understand is perhaps to cope," and finally, "Enter with doubt and exit with hope." What were some of the specific things he learned, and how did they help him?

He learned why he had so much trouble with the Christmas season and especially Christmas Eve and Day. He was always irritable, edgy and gloomy during the Christmas season, which for him lasted from Thanksgiving to the New Year. It was a miserable state for a family man like him. It was not until he shared the story of his beloved comrades being killed in an ambush on Christmas Eve – during a patrol he missed – and our exploring that with him, that the reasons for his Christmas response became clear. It was not and could not be a holiday for him. It was painfully linked to the deaths of his dearest comrades. Gaining this insight did not enable him to immediately dispel his Christmas gloom, but he was able to start to understand and control his discomfort and negative emotional response to a more substantial degree.

Walt told us once about a nasty little spat he had with his wife. They had planned a nice evening with dinner and a movie. At their favorite restaurant, the only table available was in the middle of the dining area. He found himself very reluctant to sit there. He became increasingly anxious and edgy. Finally he got up and said, "I'm leaving," not understanding why he was so upset. His wife was quite put out and snapped at him. They went home in silence, hungry.

Most combat infantrymen cannot comfortably sit in the middle of a busy restaurant. They are much more at ease sitting in the corner with a solid wall to their backs, and with a clear view of the windows and doors. Twenty to fifty years after his combat, an infantryman will not be consciously thinking about snipers shooting into the room through the windows, nor someone sneaking up and lobbing in a "potato masher" (the American nickname for the German grenade), but his conditioned combat responses are still there and he will feel uneasy unless he is situated properly.

Initially, Walt had no idea why he made this scene with his wife. He could explain it neither to her nor to himself. It was very embarrassing. I had been educated enough by my vets that I was able to suggest the connection to the "potato masher" or sniper. At first he was resistant, but as we explored it further, I could see the light go on in his eyes. He knew I was right. Those conditioned combat safety responses are never fully extinguished. But they can be successfully accommodated to, once they are remembered and made conscious. By avoiding sitting in the middle of any room, whether at school, church, a speech, a restaurant or a movie, most ex-combatants can enjoy the activity more. They need to make reservations for specific tables, get to the class or lecture in time to get the right seat, or to the cinema in time to get a good spot next to the wall with the exits in view. It also helps if they explain all this briefly to their companions. There is no shame in making this simple but effective accommodation to their past experiences.

Ex-combat infantrymen will often find themselves becoming irritable while standing in a crowd or in the open talking to someone. They might start to furtively scan their surroundings and completely miss what their companions are saying to them. When asked, they cannot explain why they do not seem to hear what their partners have been saying, or why they look edgy. They have consciously forgotten being trained to avoid open "fields of fire" (open areas easily sighted in by enemy artillery or automatic weapons), and to "not bunch up," making inviting targets for the enemy's heavy weapons. Therapy helps make these automatic responses conscious again so the here-and-now can be better explained and managed.

The cauldron of war conditions men's responses more effectively than any other training I know. These responses became automatic and fast. Many will never extinguish their startle response to sudden loud noises or to people approaching them unexpectedly from behind. It is helpful to remember that soldiers are not "weird" or "crazy" to still have these responses. They helped keep them alive and are a normal leftover from the war.

Understanding his own "anniversary responses" helps any vet cope more positively with civilian life. It helps him stay alert to unpleasant emotions that are coming from the past and complicating his efforts to live

successfully in the present. Most men have times that are uniquely troubling
to them, such as Walt's trouble with Christmas. Other men have a difficult
time which they share with most who were in a specific battle – such as
my vets who survived December 7 at Pearl Harbor, or those who made the
June landings at Normandy. In the case of Vietnam, an even larger number
of veterans become edgy and irritable as the New Year approaches, since
for many years the North Vietnamese and Vietcong launched major
offensives each Tet, their New Year's holiday.

Making the conscious connection between their dysphoric symptoms
now and the specific traumatic anniversary can radically reduce the
difficulties vets experience during their own anniversary times. They then
can take appropriate actions to better manage their responses.

One Vietnam War artilleryman, who is working fulltime as a city
manager and raising his teenage daughters as a single parent, comes in
every year in the early fall. His unit was involved in several nasty
engagements during the late fall. They provided close artillery support to
Marine reconnaissance units. He spent almost twenty months in country.
He has learned after more than a decade of intermittent therapy to see me
preventively in the early fall. He gets a little medication for sleep and
anxiety, and talks things through "one more time." He can then more
successfully cope with the increased intrusive thoughts, nightmares and
irritability. He also stops drinking and limits his caffeine intake during
those few months. In this way he avoids all the problems with fights, angry
outbursts, insomnia and fatigue that used to trouble him.

Roland, who served as a combat medic in Vietnam, grew up on a farm
in the midst of a large and loving family. His parents' anniversary was "the
most important holiday after Christmas." Post-war he became a successful
EMT, ICU nurse and finally chiropractor. He first saw me a few days after
his parents' anniversary, 30 years after Vietnam, and told me the following:

> I had already been in country several months and had been wounded twice. Our
> company began a search and destroy mission on my parents' anniversary. I
> knew I could be killed at any time and did not really expect to survive my tour.
> I thought how hard it would be on Mom and Dad and the rest of the family if I
> were killed on their anniversary. We were moving up a riverbed in a deep ravine
> when we were ambushed. As I rapidly treated the wounded, pulling several out
> of the exposed riverbed, I was praying constantly that God would spare my
> family the pain of my death on this day of all days. I was going after one last
> man, who was down in the shallow stream. I was moving in cover up the bank
> toward him, yelling at him to stay down and that I was coming. I was reaching
> out to drag him to cover when he got to his knees and looked up. My hand was

a foot from his when his face disappeared: blown off, just gone. My family was spared my death that day, but my parents' anniversary has never been the same holiday for me. I unwillingly re-experience that day in the ravine each time.

Roland has worked very effectively with his counselor. Through that work, prayer and the judicious use of a little medication, he has now drawn the sting out of this particular "anniversary reaction." He anticipates it and copes with it much better.

Several years ago Gary, another Vietnam medic, came storming into my office saying, "Doc, I'm totally losing it. I thought I was getting better, but the last few days have been hell all over again!" He was a truck driver, and he had gone to California to drop off a load and had then picked up a cargo in Fresno for a laminated wood plant in Boise. Driving home he experienced constant intrusive thoughts of Vietnam. They included powerful images of his bloodiest "dust-offs."[1] He was distressed and discouraged because he had not been this symptomatic for years. "I thought I was over most of this." We did the usual routine of discovery questions. It was summer, so it wasn't Tet-induced.

"Have you been watching anything violent?"
"Doc, you know I know better than that."
"Was there something on the news?"
"Wouldn't matter if there was because I haven't been looking or reading."
"Any bad news from family or friends? Anybody sick or dying?"
"No."
Finally I asked what he had been hauling.
"Dried blood from the slaughterhouses in Fresno."
"Dried blood? Why dried blood?"
"They use it to bind the wood panels together. They say it helps make a great glue."
"Could you smell it?"
"Hell yes! The whole frigging way!"
"Have you ever smelt it before?"
"Damn near every day in Vietnam!"

It didn't take a genius to figure out that he should never haul dried blood again. He just hadn't been able to see it because at the time all he could see, smell and think about were Vietnam "dust-offs."

Smells are one of the most powerful activators of memory. Burning hair and flesh, rotting corpses, jungles, swamps, gunpowder – all have powerful odors that can trigger a revival of combat related symptoms. Each vet has to learn his own triggers, be on guard for them, and control and manage their effects. Conscious awareness of what is happening is a key to successful coping.

One Marine from the 1st Marine Division notes that the smell of exhaust fumes, like those that came from the landing craft they used to assault beaches, still troubles him the most:

> From that day to this the heavy smell of exhaust brings back memory of the war. I can watch war movies and listen to fireworks or thunder, and they mean nothing to my memory; but the heavy smell of exhaust still makes my palms sweat ...[2]

Joe, from the 30th Infantry Division in Europe, was looking especially grim one winter. On questioning he revealed that he was having constant nightmares and even daytime intrusive thoughts of Tiger Tanks and battle scenes. As it turned out, there were three problems. It was winter, the time of his worst fighting in Europe. It was foggy, and the Germans always counterattacked in the fog because it negated our air superiority. Finally, a road crew was widening the avenue in front of his home, and they used heavy diesel equipment. The German tanks all used diesel fuel. American tanks used gasoline. After discussing these three factors, Joe concluded that the smell of diesel was the greatest disturber of his peace.

Talking through automatic responses and understanding why they are happening makes them easier to bear. The triggers continue to revive memories, and probably always will. However, often the triggers can be avoided. If they can't, then the vet's increased understanding and conscious awareness of their effects on him at least makes coping with the memories easier.

Fred, who received a battlefield commission in Korea and then was decorated multiple times for bravery in Vietnam, came in to see me for the first time after attending a granddaughter's high school basketball game:

> I could not tell you what happened in the game. I am so disgusted with myself. There was a Vietnamese-American boy who was one of the cheerleaders. A very nice young man, I am sure. He was right in front of me the whole game. Images of the war poured in. He was our cheerleader, for Christ's sake, and I actually felt like he was the enemy! How can I be thinking like that after all this time!?

Here is one of the most troubling reminders of the war for vets: people who look or sound like their previous foe. Depending on the war and the vet's experiences, a German accent or a Japanese, Korean, Arab, or Vietnamese American can provoke intrusive memories and unpleasant thoughts. The vet's war experiences have conditioned him to respond to them as the enemy.

A Korean War vet I treat went to an awards ceremony sponsored by the Korean government and supported by ours. All Korean War vets were invited to come and receive a special medal honoring their participation in the effort to keep Korea free from the tyranny of Communism. The keynote speaker was a very eloquent Korean-American politician who was fluent in Korean and English. He spoke in both languages during the ceremony, as many of the participants were Koreans who came to honor the American vets. My patient noted:

> I was comfortable whenever he was speaking English, but every time he spoke in Korean I got restless and irritable. I was disgusted with myself that after all this time just hearing Korean troubled me that much. It was a beautiful ceremony and I should have enjoyed it, but I was reminded too much of the grim experiences I had in Korea to take any pleasure in the festivities.

It can take years of frequent, peaceful exposure to undo this conditioning. Because of the unpleasant images and emotions aroused, veterans naturally avoid this exposure. The vet is left with what I call "the façade of racism." He knows Germans, Japanese and Vietnamese are real people with normal human feelings and families. He knows that in making war against them, he was killing people "just like Americans." He knows that people from Germany, Japan, Korea and Vietnam living in America are Americans. But when he sees them or hears them, his gut can still knot up and his mouth feel dry. Images of the war can intrude and he can feel threatened, as if he was in the presence of the "enemy."

These vets usually do not blame anyone but themselves. "How can I still be doing this after all this time?!" has echoed in my office many times. They talk about it, pray about it, prepare their minds for the meeting. All this can help. But it is just like all the other triggers of memory – only it can be even more intense and personal. It takes the same type of therapeutic effort and understanding to overcome this conditioned response as any other. The more the men consciously work on it and expose themselves to it, the more success they have in limiting its effects on their relationships and life.

Anniversaries, odors, sounds, news, media violence, weather, positions in buildings, people of certain races: all these and many more stimuli can be general and idiosyncratic triggers that reactivate unpleasant memories, feelings and responses connected to the war. Each veteran has to develop his own understanding of the connection between his war and the here and now. He must make conscious what has become unconscious and automatic. When he does, he gains greater freedom over his past conditioning. The war loses much of its haunting power and its ability to steal happiness from the present and future. As Walt noted, in effective treatment you "enter with doubt, exit with hope."

Notes

1   "Dust-offs" were originally unarmed air ambulance missions where the helicopter is clearly marked with a Red Cross. "Medevacs" are armed air ambulance missions. The latter became necessary because the Red Cross was not respected but instead became a high priority target for the North Vietnamese and Vietcong. According to many of my vets, later in the Vietnam War they started to mean the same thing as unarmed air ambulance missions ceased.
2   Davis op. cit. pp. 9–10.

Chapter 9

The Therapeutic Reunion

Boyd (discussed first in Chapter 4) was a Marine Corps rifleman. He had been troubled by the desecrating attitude and actions he took toward the body of a Vietcong he killed. He was also haunted by an action where he saved a Marine's life, only to "condemn him to a life worse than death":

> We had an unwritten code that we had all discussed at one time or another. If a buddy was wounded so badly that life would not be worth living, if he somehow survived, then we had agreed to let him die in the field. Problem is, I just didn't hold up my end of the bargain.
>
> Guy and I were collecting unexploded ordinance. We gave a bounty to the local Vietnamese to bring in any bombs, shells, grenades – whatever they found. This was supposed to keep the VC from getting them and turning them into booby traps. Unfortunately, they sometimes turned in stuff that had already been "fixed" by the VC. In this case it was a 105mm howitzer round. They had probably put a little wire in the arming mechanism. If you turned it just right it dropped out and exploded, but it was otherwise safe to handle. Guy was taking an armful of this ordinance to the rear of the jeep. I don't remember what I was doing, but I was up front. As he placed it into the jeep bed, the 105mm round exploded. I was knocked down but unhurt. As I ran to Guy I saw our medic run the opposite direction. Guy's right leg was completely gone from mid-thigh down. His left leg was mangled and shredded. The right stump was gushing blood from the femoral artery like a garden hose. My adrenalin was pumping in full combat mode as I encircled the right stump with both hands and squeezed with all the strength I possessed. The bleeding stopped from the right stump, but there was nothing I could do about the left leg, as it took both hands and all the force I could exert to control the bleeding from the right.
>
> It seemed like an eternity but must have been only moments when the medic returned. He put a ligature over the right stump so I could release it. As we worked on his left leg and other wounds, Guy regained consciousness. He seemed unaware of what had happened to his legs. His right hand was sliced in half, with only his thumb and index finger remaining. He raised his hand and showed it to me, saying, "No one will ever want a guy with a hand like this." A few minutes later a medevac [helicopter] arrived.

A few days later Boyd was wounded and subsequently decorated for bravery for saving a South Vietnamese soldier's life in a firefight. He was flown to the same hospital as Guy. "I tried to see him, but he was in intensive care the whole time and they wouldn't let me. I learned, though, that they had amputated his left leg. It was too mangled to save. He was then taken to the States." Boyd never saw Guy again nor heard what finally happened to him. "I was afraid to find out. I was afraid that he had lived and his life was hell and that I was responsible for keeping a buddy alive I should have let die."

I had treated Boyd on and off for years, but only in a limited way, as he lived 300 miles from our VA hospital. We had developed a good relationship but had made no progress on this issue before he was admitted to our intensive residential PTSD treatment program. This program brought a handful of combat vets together in a residential setting for intensive group and individual trauma treatment. It usually admitted vets like Boyd who lived hundreds of miles from Boise and had limited access to this type of care.

Boyd's inpatient therapist began focusing on this issue involving Guy. She finally convinced Boyd to try to contact him. It worked. Boyd had not yet completed the program when he contacted Guy by phone. Guy responded by driving immediately to Boise. I was there for the reunion and for a few years participated in several follow-up meetings. Guy and Boyd would both drive to Boise about every three months. They would spend a day together and then meet in my office to work on issues, with me acting as "coach" for those sessions. In reality I did little more than listen. I knew I was privileged to be an honored guest for these reunions.

Guy's own story was remarkable. He had been treated initially at the Philadelphia Naval Hospital where there was a specialized unit for amputees. "With God's help and some great work from the staff there, I finally accepted the challenge to live life to its fullest. I got out of bed and stopped feeling sorry for myself. I found God at a deeper level. My faith sustains me to this day." Guy was chief of prosthetics at a VAMC in a neighboring state when he got Boyd's phone call and drove to Boise for that first remarkable reunion. He has been helping other paralyzed and limbless vets adapt and thrive since Vietnam.

As I watched Boyd and Guy work together over the next few years, I marveled at the therapeutic and healing power for both men of this remarkable reunion. Nothing heals the soul's pain quite like being in the presence of someone you love and respect, and who loves and respects you. Quiet, deep love and respect radiated from their eyes and infused every gesture. Even "the invited guest" felt nurtured. One of the benefits of engaging in this type of work is that every successful therapy seems in some small way to heal the therapist too.

Boyd and Guy first replayed the events of the war they shared together. Now as mature adults, they could look back and together shine greater light and understanding on what happened to them as teenage warriors. For instance, Boyd had always been critical of the medic who initially seemed to run away, leaving him in the helpless position of holding the bleeding stump of Guy's right leg in his hands. Should he release it or not? What if the enemy appeared? How could he defend them both without letting Guy die? Guy was going to die anyway from his wounds if something else wasn't done soon. Holding that leg stump was not enough, but it was all he could do. Talking together, they began to exonerate the medic. First, he returned. Second, he brought his kit with him so he could actually do something useful like tie off the arteries. Criticism turned to respect, and a man was forgiven in absentia. Boyd's feelings changed from blaming anger toward the medic to forgiveness and respect. Forgiving someone else always makes it easier to accept forgiveness and love from others.

Humor was always present in these meetings. Horrors were laughed at and made smaller. Questions were answered. Yes, Guy did not initially realize he had lost both legs. And yes, for a while he blamed Boyd for saving him. And most important, "Was Guy sorry Boyd and the medic had saved him?" "Absolutely Not!" He had lived a good life. And the glory of the good life he had lived was laid out in sufficient, healing detail so that Boyd could take some pride in having saved Guy. They shared the intimacy of their spiritual quests and the strength they had received from God. They reinforced each other's positive efforts to cope. They looked at how they could help others.

Guy, who had previously avoided significant engagement in treatment with mental health professionals, found this reunion just as healing as Boyd:

Before the reunion with Boyd I was still denying that the war troubled me emotionally in any significant way. Because of the trust and respect I had for Boyd, I listened when Boyd said, "I think you have PTSD also." With that comment Boyd kicked the bloody door open – ushering me into my own treatment. Every part of this reunion process that was helpful to him helped me in a similar way. I had to face the pain of the losses I had experienced and shed many tears of deep grief. My therapist had to say to me more than once, "Nobody has ever cried to death." He was right, but I struggled to believe him at first. I was slow to accept the truth that exploring the traumatic past of the war could help me heal; but it has. I thank God for Boyd's help in Vietnam and now as well.

Just a few months ago Roland, the medic in the previous chapter who survived the ambush on his parent's anniversary, brought his wife to my office. They told me of the remarkable reunion they had just had with Roland's former company commander:

> He was an excellent officer. We all loved and respected him. He was tough, brave and savvy. We were ambushed as our company proceeded up a valley. I was in the command group when we were hit by rocket-propelled grenades and small arms fire. The captain, executive officer, and both CP radiomen were wounded. A piece of shrapnel shattered the captain's right arm. He was still directing our defense over the field radio as I tried to treat him. He was dying before my eyes as blood poured from his brachial artery. I could not get it clamped or get the bleeding stopped with pressure. Under intense fire and desperate, I removed the lace from his boot, looped it around his shoulder at the armpit, stood up, and placing my boot on his shoulder, cinched the lace as tight as I could. He groaned, showered me with curses, and nearly passed out from the pain. He had lost so much blood I feared his veins had collapsed, but amazingly I was able to hit a vein and start plasma on my first try. When I got him on the medevac, he was nearly unconscious and so pale and weak I was sure he would die. I felt I had failed to save the most important man in the company. He became part of that list of men I should have saved.

In my office Roland continued with the story of the here and now:

> Doc, as I mentioned to you a few months ago I read in a history of some of our actions, quotes from a captain who had the same last name as my Captain, who I thought was dead. I then called our unit historian who gave me this man's address. I did not think he was my Captain but I had to know, so I wrote him a brief note asking him if was my CO, and had truly lived when I thought he had died. Four days after mailing the letter he called and we spoke on the phone. The first words he said to me were, "Oh my God, I can't believe I'm talking to the man who saved my life!" He immediately put me at ease. It was wonderful to know he was actually alive! Since my wife and I were going cross-country, we stopped at the Captain's insistence and spent two days there. He and his wife were so gracious and welcoming. He told us the rest of his story.
>
> The Captain knew he was dying on the medevac because he remembers feeling his life force flowing from his body and wanting to stop breathing. But he did not want the enemy to have the satisfaction of killing him. To keep himself alive he counted rivets on the chopper roof and made himself breathe

every fifth rivet. He was eventually stabilized in Vietnam and brought to Fitzsimmons Army Hospital in Denver. His wife came to see him, spent an hour with him, left, and filed for divorce, saying she wasn't living with a man without an arm. He was feeling very low when a Red Cross worker started coming by to talk and try to cheer him up. They drew close over the next several months and have now been married almost 30 years. He stayed in the army but could not be a line officer without a right arm. He earned a masters degree in hospital administration and an MBA, and ended up serving as a hospital administrator and director. He just retired as a full colonel.

Roland continued: "We caught up on each others' lives and families. We rehashed a lot of our experiences in Vietnam and discussed the men with whom we served and what had happened to them. Finally, the day we left he gave me this." Roland opened a box and brought out a beautiful reproduction sculpture of two men. One is lying on the ground, wounded. The other is a medic kneeling next to him, treating his wounds. A rifle, stuck bayonet first in the ground, has a bottle of plasma taped to its butt as it drips into the soldier's vein. A fresh inscription had been added to the base of the sculpture that read, "Doc, thanks for saving my life."

In the office all three of us are moved to tears of joy. This is therapy of the best sort. Roland can never think of Vietnam again without remembering this reunion. No other treatment could be more effective.

Reunions are rarely quite this dramatic and powerful, but when they do occur they are almost always healing. It is as if they give the original events a new and healthier meaning. They often bring at least some clarity, peace and release. In the case of both Boyd and Roland, their reunions infused their war experiences with a saving grace of personal redemption. Because they were there and took forceful action, a man lived. Not only did a man live, he lived well. And it wasn't just any man. It was in each case a dearly beloved comrade. This type of experience in the here and now begins to free the vet from the tyranny of twisted negative thoughts about all his combat horrors and the negative image of self they can induce. Here in Guy and the Captain was incontrovertible evidence that Boyd and Roland did something noble and worthwhile in their war. They simply cannot think about the war any longer without thinking about these positive events.

Richard Peterson, PhD, wrote a refreshing book about his own redemptive voyage. It describes his experiences as a teenager in a newly formed American division that was sent to guard the line in an "inactive area of the front" in the Ardennes in early December 1944. A week later this completely green outfit was surrounded as the Germans launched their fierce offensive at the beginning of the Battle of the Bulge. They fought off the Germans until they had no more ammunition and then became POWs. They were imprisoned under harsh circumstances – finally being freed in May 1945.

Speaking of his return home and the effects of his wartime trauma on his subsequent life, he explains:

> Life followed a pattern laid out while I was a teenager: university, marriage, children, career, all of which reflected outward success. However, I lived in a personal life of desperation. Intimacy did not exist within my family. I made the whole process of living tolerable with the numbing help of alcohol. How the rest of my family endured life with me I did not know or, at times, care. Innocent children never knew their father. The longtime marriage ended in divorce. My career, built up over 20 years, ended in dismissal, my father died and I found myself working in another town at half capacity. Always alone and trapped inside a mental barbed wire enclosure, life was tiresome at best. Finally, alcohol no longer offered escape and I had to give up completely.[1]

Peterson discusses his finding God and sobriety while being treated in a VA hospital for his alcoholism. He then went on to get a PhD in psychology and, as part of his own therapy, helped to organize and attended the first reunion of his division in Oklahoma in 1988. Speaking of that reunion he notes, "During the three days we were together, it seemed we never stopped talking. There is no question we all felt a release of old pressures."[2] He goes on to describe the sharing and confessing and supportive listening that went on at that and subsequent reunions. They even returned to Germany together to the town of their captivity and had a reunion with the townspeople and some of their surviving guards. All this furthered the process of healing, forgiveness and recovery.

Bob had been in therapy with me nearly three years when I was able to observe firsthand the deep healing that came from his special reunion. Bob joined the US Army prior to Pearl Harbor. He was aboard ship in San Francisco Bay in 1941 when an attack of appendicitis hospitalized him. His unit sailed for the Philippines without him. They were the last unit to get there before the war started. Very few survived the early battles and subsequent captivity when the Philippines fell to the Japanese.

After recovering from his appendectomy, Bob was assigned to a glider unit. Gliders were loaded with troops and supplies, towed behind transport planes, and then released behind enemy lines to land in the battle zone. Bob's outfit would go in with the gliders to repair and recover them for reuse.

In September 1944, the C-47 towing his glider unit was damaged by anti-aircraft fire and crash landed outside Best, a small town near Eindhoven, Holland, about 20 miles behind German lines. They had come there with the 101st Airborne Division to assist in the capture of several key bridges. He was involved in intense combat as they held their positions against German counterattacks until their unit was transferred out in January 1945.

They had been on the ground just outside Best about one week. It was Sunday morning and the local townspeople had finished Mass and were coming out to visit them when Bob heard an explosion about 100 yards away that sounded like a German 88mm artillery shell, followed by screams and calls for help. He and three of his friends took bandages and a medical kit and rushed to the scene to find three little girls ages seven, nine and 11 dreadfully wounded. The 11-year-old had one eye blown out, and they all seemed to be bleeding from "100 shrapnel wounds each." The soldiers rapidly began treating and bandaging the girls. They knew the girls would die if they did not get them quickly to skilled help. Their unit commander agreed to let them drive the girls, in the unit's only functioning jeep, to the Catholic hospital in Eindhoven, five miles away. One man drove and the three others each held a girl in their arms as they rushed to the hospital – risking being shelled by the Germans the whole way. Bob had put a compress over the 11-year-old's shattered eye socket and tried to comfort her as he cradled her in his arms until they arrived at the hospital and turned them over to the Dutch medical staff.

Bob and the men in his unit formed a deep bond with these girls and their families. They visited them as often as the fighting allowed and shared their rations with them. "Our supply situation was desperate, but what we had we shared." Talking with the surgeons at the hospital, Bob discovered that they were trying to arrange for a specialist to come from Switzerland to repair the girl's eye socket and construct an attractive prosthesis. The cost was a prohibitive $3000. No one had that type of money, but Bob had just won a pot nearly that large in a crapshoot. He planned on using what he had won to cover the cost of the surgery, but when the rest of the unit got wind of his plans they refused to let him do it alone and all contributed equally, giving the entire sum to the hospital to pay for the surgery and the prosthesis. Bob also bought all three girls beautiful dresses to wear when they were finally discharged from the hospital.

Bob wondered what happened to the three girls, but he had no more contact with them or their families after being transferred away in January 1945. Bob had been in therapy with me a few years in 1994 when he received a call from a retired Dutch artillery officer. The officer invited him to stay in his home for a week in September as all of Holland celebrated their liberation by American and British forces from the Nazis in the fall of 1944. The Dutch government paid for the airfare of every surviving member of the 101st and 82nd Airborne Divisions and all associated troops who made the air assaults in Operation Market Garden, the code-name given to this battle. A Dutch family hosted each man who accepted the invitation to come. Two of my vets attended, including Bob. Bob's host refused to allow him to spend any of his own money.

Prior to his arrival in Holland, Bob's Dutch host asked him if he had any special requests for his visit. Bob told him about his experience with the three girls and their families and mentioned he would like to visit them if they were still alive. Bob had been in Holland three days when his host's wife said she wanted to take him to a nearby museum. They did not go to the museum but went instead to a surprise gathering of the families of these three girls. Two of the three girls were still alive and had children and grandchildren. The seven-year-old girl had died of a cerebral aneurysm at age 19.

Bob was glowing with happiness when he returned to Boise and described the event in these words:

> It was a joyous and deeply moving reunion. People gave their hearts to us and we responded in kind. It opened my heart up to a new happiness. Those girls' families were wonderful. I even met some Germans whose relatives had been killed in that battle. They didn't hold no grudges. The whole experience really helped me feel more peace about my war experiences.

In 1998 the son of the woman who had been wounded at age nine brought her to Boise to visit Bob. The son had just retired as a sea captain. He rented a car and took his mother and Bob on a week-long tour of the western US. It reinforced the happiness and peace engendered in Bob by the original reunion in 1994.

I have marveled over the years as I have seen the therapeutic benefits of reunions unfold before my eyes. In addition to those cases already discussed, I have watched a vet seek out the surviving members of his bomber crew. I have seen the healing effects of another man's yearly gatherings with his WWII aircrew, ever since his retirement 20 years ago. Others have gone to unit reunions and celebrations. They all bear the same kind of positive fruit. Memories are processed and better understood. Friendships are reaffirmed. Grief is displayed and processed. Hearts are eased. Old hurts can be tempered and soothed. The exact nature of the therapeutic benefits depends on the men and current and previous circumstances, but there appears always to be some benefit.

I now recognize that even those who have lost their comrades can benefit from a type of reunion. I have seen it as men visit the Vietnam Memorial and find special names on The Wall and commune with their departed spirits, finding some solace. I see it as men write their memoirs and evoke the memories of those long dead, and seem to arrive at a greater peace. I have been taught by these experiences to ask about and suggest contact with old comrades. I encourage the visiting of museums, memorials and graveyards. Finally, I recognize that the group therapy process itself provides a type of therapeutic reunion as one of its healing forces. The men in group can become surrogates for those in their original units who are now gone or unavailable. As in the case of Herb in Chapter 6, they are able to confess to the group and receive absolution if that is what they need. They are heard by those who have a true sense of what they faced and can fully empathize and share in return. They can mourn together with deep understanding.

Notes

1   Peterson, Richard, PhD., *Healing the Child Warrior: A Search for Inner Peace*, p. 102.
2   Ibid p. 104.

Chapter 10

"Keeping the Demons at Bay": Sharing and Support and "Working Through" in Group Therapy

"Where no counsel is, the people fall: but in the multitude of counselors there is safety."

Proverbs 11:14

When I started treating Doug years ago, I was sure he was psychotic. His soul seemed at war. He told me he prayed constantly to try to "keep the demons at bay." He felt that at any time, without God's help, they might overwhelm him. He occasionally reported a smell "like sulfur or smoke" when they were around. He reported being haunted at night by scenes from Hell. He never got more than a few hours of sleep. At times he felt if he slept, "they will get me for sure." "That's one reason I used to drink so much. But I finally saw that alcohol was no answer, so I stopped." More than once he remarked, "Sometimes prayer is all I have to keep me going." I knew he had fought in Korea but he did not appear to want to talk about it and I did not push.

I learned early on in this work that if combat vets were also psychotic, I ran a high risk of making the psychosis worse by trying to get them to talk about their war trauma. I couldn't take them into a combat support group either. I have seen them break down and start floridly hallucinating as other group members began talking about their war experiences in meaningful detail.

I treated Doug with anti-psychotic meds for what I thought were his hallucinations. He admitted the meds "took the edge off," but they never fully made the "demons" go away. Antidepressants and sleep meds helped a little also. He acknowledged that he was afraid that if he told me too much, "I might lock him up." After a decade of seeing me he began to share a little more about Korea, including some of the horrors of "finishing off wounded Chinese who begged for mercy with their eyes." I had the surprising sense that unlike most combat vets who had developed psychoses, it seemed to help Doug to confess these horrors to me. These events also seemed to be tied in with why he felt "unforgivable."

By this time my first WWII combat vets group was overflowing, with 15 men enrolled. Two were "snowbirds" and spent the winters in Arizona, but the others attended every session. In the summer there was no more space in the room. That group had existed for eight years, and I had rarely seen a therapy group work so well. I called it the WWII group because most of the men were WWII vets; but there were some who fought in WWII and Korea, one who served in Korea only, and one master sergeant who spent two years with the 5th Special Forces in Vietnam and had also served as a teenager in Korea.

In a period of two months I received six more referrals. My co-therapist and I agreed we could not add any more to the current group, so we started a second group. Within a month we had nine attending. This group had an even mix of WWII, Korean and older Vietnam vets. The Vietnam vets were the age of the Korean vets and had been involved in Special Forces-type units. This new group was starting to gel.

At the same time, Doug was talking more and more about Korea. He seemed more stable than he had been in years. He was taking his meds and keeping all his appointments. We discussed group therapy. He wanted to try it. I had seen it do such remarkable things for these older vets that I agreed to let him join, under the stipulation that if either he or I thought it was making him worse, he would stop immediately. A quiet and sincere man who had served as a rifleman and noncom in the worst Korea had to offer, Doug was readily accepted by the other men in the new group.

Doug had been in group a few weeks when Dave came with his Samurai sword and told his grim tale of "battlefield justice" in all its detail, right down to executing two Japanese with the sword (see Chapter 4). I was closely observing Doug's response for signs of increasing psychosis, but surprisingly this event seemed to help him. Six months into group, Doug was thinking and speaking more clearly and was using much less medication! This miserably isolated man was making friends with the other men. They were reaching out to him. He was regularly bringing candy and cookies to share. He began gingerly to reveal what haunted him most. He fully engaged in treatment, often leading us into crucial discussions. He stopped looking psychotic to me. I asked him privately and then in group what was happening. This is what he said: "These men are heroes. They are heroes because it is harder to live well after the war than to have died in it. They have helped me change my attitude. I listen and learn. They were willing to die for those they love. That is like what Christ did." Referring to the men in the group, he would often quietly quote the Bible: "Greater love hath no man than this, that a man lay down his life for his friends."[1] He summed it all up by saying, "These men have become my counselors and are showing me the way." Two weeks later he gave me the reference from Proverbs quoted at this chapter's beginning.

What I saw happening was that an isolated and withdrawn man, lost in the horrors of his war, began to make real connections with other men. These connections gave him understanding and hope. His perspective changed and so did mine. I had interpreted his "living hell" as a psychosis. Although I still believe he is vulnerable to psychosis, through the mutual sharing and support of group therapy, his Hell became more clearly the continued hell of the Korean War echoing in his life and his own battle for redemption from what he had gone through. The demons were, in reality, the haunting and common images of war. The smell of "sulfur" was the odor of gunpowder. His religious perspective seemed to be transformed into a power for healing rather than a "losing battle with Satan." For Doug this was some of the fruit of meaningful sharing and support.

Doug also benefited from a therapeutic process called "working through." Working through is an ill-defined but essential therapeutic process, embracing all the therapeutic processes we have discussed so far. It is a recursive process that begins with the patient refining and deepening his understanding of what happened in the war and how those events are affecting him now. Then he puts that understanding to use in his life. He practices thinking and living differently. As he tries to act on what he has learned in the first stages of therapy, he deepens his understanding of the effects of war on his life. This deepened understanding leads to more action and practice, resulting in further insight and then more action. This cycle of healthy change is what we call working through. It involves a change of heart and outlook that is strong enough to lead to a healthier life. It embodies mental, emotional, social and spiritual work that spring from a new perspective or fresh look at life. The 12 Steps of Alcoholics Anonymous and the idea of repentance in some religions are closely related concepts.

Working through is independent of group therapy and takes place in many forums, but it is always an important part of any successful group therapy. Working through is part of why reunions heal, as the men process their memories together and gain deeper insight into what happened to them in the war and how it affects them now in their maturity. It occurs in successful individual and couples therapy as those involved refine and practice what they are discovering in the course of therapy.

It occurs when people attempt to write truthfully and meaningfully about themselves. It has been happening to me as a therapist as I write and think about what I have experienced and learned working with vets over the last 20 years.

Working through occurs in every good autobiography about war I have read. Even many of the book titles evoke it: *Good-bye Darkness, With the Old Breed from Pelelieu to Okinawa, Reach for the Sky, The Men of Company K, Healing the Child Warrior, Pacific War Diary, To Hell and Back, Out of the Night, The Other Side of Time, Fly for Your Life*, and *Man's Search for Meaning*. These titles evoke images of new perspectives, meaningful reflection, movement towards light, respectful fellowship and redemption.

The group process is an ideal forum for the working through process. Vets do it together and benefit from participating in each other's healing. Sometimes poetry describes it best, as you can see in this poem written by a member of a combat support group led by one of my co-workers:

Group
Twenty-three years
after the war
they recount the
stories like
beads on a rosary,
one by one, as if
checking inventory in
the stockroom.
The charred memories
wind round the room
flowing like thick
black smoke on a
phantom evening breeze
off the South China Sea.
Someone will say,
"There isn't much
to say," and talk
nonstop for 15
minutes, unaware,
while the others
think to themselves
"I thought I
was the only one."
They touch their own

> pain in one another's
> memories, gingerly,
> holding their souls
> overhead with both
> hands while wading through
> a river of silent years.
> Their lives are lists
> of broken moments,
> large and small
> tragedies piled angrily
> like the rubble aftermath of
> an artillery barrage.
> They search for new
> memories to store beside the
> old – a weights and measures
> system of stability and
> growth, a way to move on,
> to let the stories rest
> like respected friends at
> peace, though not forgotten.
> – Dan Koper

The poet has used phrases that perfectly express key healing processes in group therapy. "Charred memories wind round the room flowing ..." so accurately describes the rhythm of therapy and sharing that occurs in dynamic, healthy groups. When the group is functioning well, the therapist just watches silently as the healthy sharing unfolds.

"Someone ... will ... talk ... while others think ... 'I thought I was the only one'" grasps the therapeutic essence of discovering that you are not alone in your suffering and soul searching. Others struggle with the same issues. This lightens the individual's private burden. A shared burden is always easier to bear.

"They touch their own pain in another's memories ..." Initially the vet's own story can sometimes be too overwhelming and painful when he first tries to share it. He cannot understand and process it effectively. But when another talks and he listens with his heart, he can begin to recognize and name his own pain and gain greater understanding.

"Gingerly holding their souls overhead ..." It is delicate soul work. Entered into with great caution. Move slowly. Pause. Listen.

"They search for ... a way to move on, to let the stories rest like respected friends at peace ..." That is the goal and hope: stories told, worked through, and now laid at rest because of the therapeutic labor.

Let me share with you the flow of a group session from a few years ago. I wrote this down immediately after the conclusion of the group:

We began as I asked Doug why he looked so troubled. He admitted he has been having suicidal thoughts on and off and feeling very unworthy. He has been ruminating over some of his Korean War experiences. When he arrived he was sent immediately to the front to a hardened and bloody unit. They had just taken a hill back from the Chinese. He was ordered to go out with others and make sure all the Chinese were dead. If not, they were to finish them off. He killed badly wounded Chinese then and on subsequent occasions. On guard duty much later he shot a Chinese who approached in the night. Now he wonders if the soldier was trying to surrender or defect. He said he would never know for sure, but the man did not have a weapon on him when checked in the morning. He recounted the many years of alcohol abuse he went through after the war. Finally he found Christ again and got sober, but he has never felt forgiven for what he did in Korea. He knows he needs God but fears approaching Him.

When he finished, there was a pause. Then Bill spoke. He fought in Korea and then served six tours of six months each in Vietnam and Southeast Asia as a special operative, often on missions behind enemy lines. He told about being captured and held by his three captors in a bamboo tiger cage. He asked for water. He explained that the word for water and urine are closely related in Vietnamese, but he spoke the language well and asked for it clearly and politely. His three captors responded by coming and peeing all over him and laughing. When they had captured him, he had been searched, but they missed the string saw and garrote he had sewn into the seam of his pants. That night while the three guards slept, he used the string saw to quietly saw through his cage. He garroted and knifed the three guards in their sleep. He searched them and found pictures of their wives and children. He often wonders why he did not just slip away in the dark. Was he so full of hate that he risked the time to kill them just because they pissed all over him?

There was another pause. Then Larry, a retired US Special Forces officer, spoke of leading a unit of former Vietcong. They had become disenchanted with their corrupt VC leaders, defected and were then recruited by the CIA to fight for us. He had been fighting in Southeast Asia for over a year. He was asked by a new "hot dog" regular Army Lt. Colonel to take his team into an area held by the VC and North Vietnamese and do a recon. In this particular region there were only two sites suitable for direct helicopter landings due to the rugged terrain and deep jungle. Larry responded that it would be suicide to use either site because the enemy would have both spots covered with heavy weapons. He said if the colonel's superiors really needed the area checked out, Larry's team could fly to the rocky scrub several miles away, rappel in, and go on foot to scope out potential targets. This would take a few days and be difficult, but it would involve much less risk. The colonel refused, asking how he could possibly know the VC would be ready to ambush an insertion. They continued to argue, and finally Larry stomped off in disgust.

The colonel went to another Special Forces unit led by a lieutenant with less experience and made the same request. When Larry heard that the lieutenant had agreed to the mission, he went to him to try to talk him out of it. During the conversation the lieutenant implied that my patient had been there too long, had lost his nerve, and was too cautious. At that Larry left, frustrated and deeply concerned. The mission went forward. All four helicopters were shot down and every man killed. Larry was then ordered to lead a mission to recover the bodies. They needed a full-scale attack with several gun ships providing suppressive fire to get in and out, and they still lost more men. Many of the original men had been killed in their plastic seats and in the ensuing fires were fused to them. Larry's team had to cut them apart to get them out. It was the single most heart-rending mission of his career.

For a long time he carried a murderous rage towards the colonel. Then as he went over the whole affair in his mind, he eventually decided that he was the one most at fault. He had the most experience. He knew it was a suicide mission, yet because his pride had been wounded by certain remarks, he let them go without going to all the lengths he could to stop them. He feels now that he could eventually have persuaded them to do the mission correctly. He feels some of their blood is on his hands.

Larry ended by talking about an incident in which his unit ambushed a VC assassination team. The VC leader had been wounded, and then as he tried to flee, had fallen on a pointed stake, planted as part of the preparations for the ambush. He was still alive when they found him. Their medic confirmed that the VC could not be saved. Larry ordered his ex-VC lieutenant to shoot him. He refused, saying he would not kill a helpless man. It was against his religion. Larry finally went up and shot the wounded man in the head to put him out of his misery.

There was another longer pause. I spoke of two other vets I had treated in another setting, one who blamed himself for mercifully ending the life of a mortally wounded American, and the other who blamed himself for not having the guts to finish off three Americans who were dying in great pain and could not be rescued. After another period of silence I wondered aloud what the spirits of all these terribly wounded men would say now about those who had put them out of their misery. Did anyone believe they would blame their merciful executioners now? After another pause Doug, who had spoken first about his experiences in Korea, whispered he didn't think they would. I wondered aloud, if they could forgive him now, why could not his God? Nothing more was said, and for that day the group ended.

You have to understand that this is "... holding their souls overhead with both hands while wading through a river of silent years." This is "touching their own pain in another's memories ..." This is discovering that "I am not the only one." In telling these stories to each other, the men share their hearts and souls. They reveal their pain to help one another. Groups like this do not spring up overnight. It sometimes takes years of careful tending and trust building to get there. The men have to fully trust each other and their therapists.

Good group therapy often follows this pattern. We start on one topic – killing the wounded – we wind through various kinds of killing and end up where we started – killing the wounded. In the process various facets of the meaning of war killings are explored. The men involved touch their memories and plumb some of their deepest feelings. There is also much pondering and feeling going on by the men who are not talking. It takes patience, openness and consistency to get to this point; and once there, delicacy is needed. The therapist needs to say little if anything at this stage.

These men were deep in the "working through" process. In addition to the three men who spoke most in the session related above, we had a 1st Marine Division vet who survived the horrors of Pelelieu and Okinawa; two more who survived Guadalcanal; a forward artillery observer who saw death in every form with the 79th Division in Europe; an 82nd Airborne paratrooper who made all their airdrops starting with Normandy; a Marine who spent two years as a gunner on the carrier *Enterprise* in the South Pacific and a WWII army medic. Another member received a battlefield commission in Korea and then flew choppers in Vietnam. Finally, there were two WWII US Army riflemen, one who served in Okinawa and one who fought in Burma.

The men in these groups keep sharing and working. They excavate the past and follow the threads of its effects on the present. They mutually support each other's efforts to move on positively. They rejoice in one another's successes and comfort each other in loss. They expand their group work well beyond the formal group therapy time. By the time my co-therapist and I arrive to conduct the group sessions, these men have been meeting for over an hour. They chat as they eat lunch together in the VA canteen. They are always talking and sharing when we arrive for group, and they leave group together still visiting. Several drive together to the VA. One WWII vet, Ken, puts it this way: "I think this group has helped me more than anything. It is just like I was back in the Company. I have been able to get close to these men just like my war buddies." They will be done with their therapy when they decide it is over. A few die, like Herb, having found a measure of peace. Others, troubled to the point they finally seek help, will replace them.

Before we explore other topics, it is important to understand that formal group therapy conducted by a therapist is not the only type of group therapy that treats combat-related symptoms effectively. Many informal but deeply healing therapy groups are formed spontaneously as ex-combatants make relationships with other combat vets from their families and in their post-war workplaces. One of the most effective settings for this is the military itself.

Roland's Captain from the previous chapter illustrates this as dramatically as any man could. Recently he and his wife came to visit Roland and his wife, and all four came to see me. We shared two hours together as the Captain elucidated for me just how healing and effective this type of naturalistic group therapy can be.

For the Captain it began in his family. His grandfather had served in WWI. His father and uncles had all fought in WWII. He saw Vietnam as "an opportunity to join the fraternity of civilian warriors" in his family. As his time of service approached, his surviving relatives shared many of their combat experiences with him to prepare him for what he would experience, and to help him avoid mistakes they had made. This included telling him of times "they had experienced the sorrow of having made wrong choices in battle." They shared all they had experienced to help him learn from their successes and their failures. He learned from them and his ROTC leaders who were also ex-combatants that "it is never worth the personal cost of breaking the boundaries of our cultural and Christian ethics just to achieve a brief tactical or strategic advantage."

This pre-war "group therapy" left him committed to fighting an "ethical war" and helping his men do the same so they could all live the rest of their lives without deep regrets:

> As a company commander I did my duty and we fought to win but I also did all I could to keep my men alive and get them home squared away so they could live with themselves the rest of their lives. At times I had to bullshit my superiors to avoid getting my men hurt to accomplish nothing. Many times we risked our lives and gave the enemy brief tactical advantages to avoid civilian casualties, but it was worth it in the end. On one occasion the VC used a screen of women and children to cause us to hold our fire and enable them to gain fire superiority over us. My men risked their lives by leaving cover to get those women and children to safety. Once they had accomplished this, they responded to the enemy with the most effective and courageous assault I have ever seen to regain the battle advantage and drive the VC from the battlefield.
>
> To the limit of my power, I kept my men from committing anything they would later regret that did not involve killing the enemy. On one patrol three of

my men shot up a water buffalo for sport. First I gave them a brutal verbal lashing. Then I made them find the owner and pay him. Finally they spent hours in the hot sun, digging a hole with their entrenching tools large enough to bury that huge animal. I never had another man in my company do anything like that again.

The Captain did make mistakes. Many of his men did get killed and wounded, and he killed the enemy himself. He was evacuated from combat with a wound that resulted in the total loss of his right arm, 26 months as a patient, and the end of his first marriage. How did he cope with this successfully after the war?

He met a Red Cross worker who never let him feel sorry for himself and eventually married him. He worked hard to recover from the loss of his right arm and to make the military a career. The senior combatants in his family continued to process his and their war experiences with him. Toward the end of his time in rehabilitation, he began serving as the executive officer of a medical unit made up almost entirely of Vietnam combat medics and medical personnel serving the last few months of their enlistments before discharge. This unit was a problem for all their previous commanders because of their resistance to stateside US Army discipline and "spit and polish." He explains how he successfully approached leading these ex-combatants:

> I recognized that all they wanted was to do something meaningful. I found meaningful things for them to do rather than the usual Army nonsense. The result was a radical improvement in morale and appearance. It caught the eye of my superiors and they found a place for a one-armed officer as a unit commander in the medical corps. It was about then that I started organizing my own version of what the Army called "hip pocket" training.
>
> I had learned from my family and combat seasoned ROTC officers how important it was for the old warriors to teach the young soldiers what war was like so they could fight effectively and ethically. I got together with the other ex-combatants in every unit I led the rest of my career and organized unit training based specifically on our wartime experiences. Each combatant would turn all his experiences, whether good or bad, into training sessions that would help the green troops learn from the experiences of those who had already faced combat. Many of our worst experiences became our most effective training tools. For the experienced as well as the uninitiated, this was the most popular and effective training we did.

The Captain participated in the best type of group therapy possible over the whole course of his military career. He continued to work through and process even his worst failures as he used them to teach others. He participated in many of the military's humanitarian missions. He kept his units busy doing meaningful service and meaningful training no matter where they were stationed.

This type of extended "group therapy" and service is a good recipe for successful post-war adjustment. Occasionally I encounter other vets who have followed a similar path to a successful post-war adjustment by establishing long-term, supportive relationships with other ex-combatants in their families and among their co-workers – relationships that foster the healing that comes from meaningful sharing and support and working through.

Note

1   Bible, John 15:13, KJV.

Chapter 11

Humor

I have no idea who first said, "Laughter is the best medicine,"[1] but they knew what they were talking about. Sometimes it is the only medicine. Humor has the ability to lighten the mood. It can make the unbearable bearable. It can reframe in a more positive way even the most negative experiences. It can open our minds to new perspectives, new approaches to problems, and new solutions.

When Dale first came to see me, it was not by his choice. He had been receiving medication for years from his family physician to help him sleep and manage his nighttime anxiety. Although this was a drug usually prescribed by psychiatrists, he had never seen one. When his family physician died, he decided that rather than find a new one, he would come to the VA for his care. The internist assigned to him at our hospital said, "I'll be happy to prescribe this for you as long as Dr. Dewey says it is OK." He was sent to see me, and we hit it off well. He had been in the 82nd Airborne Division and had dropped on Normandy and Nijmegen and then fought near St. Vith in the Battle of the Bulge. At both Normandy and Nijmegen, over two thirds of his company was wounded, captured, or killed. At St. Vith almost half became casualties. He went through it all unscathed. He gave me *Band of Brothers* by Stephen Ambrose to further my education, saying, "They weren't my outfit but what they went through was just how it was for us." He readily entered into group therapy saying: "I should have found you guys a long time ago."

Dale had stopped smoking eight years earlier when his first lung was removed because of lung cancer. One month after joining group he was diagnosed with cancer in his second lung. There was no treatment, let alone a cure. He was told he had less than six months to live. When I asked him how he was doing, he responded with the following joke:

> Well, Doc, it's like this. A window washer was cleaning windows from a scaffold outside the top floor of the Empire State Building. A sudden gust of wind knocked him off and his safety belt snapped. As he was passing the 65th floor a man leaned out and called, "How ya doing?" He yelled back, "All right so far." Doc that is just how I am doing – all right so far.

He told at least one joke every group and kept us laughing until he died. Whenever anyone asked how he was holding up, it was "all right so far." And if we gave him time, he would tell another joke.

I believe Dale lost his fear of death in 1944 and 1945. He had faced death often, fighting desperately against the Germans. Falling from the top of a building was not unlike the parachute drops he made behind enemy lines into enemy fire. He felt he beat the odds many times to survive WWII. He seemed to feel that every day he had since then was a bonus and he was going to enjoy each one as long as they lasted. He did not let worries about a future he could not change steal happiness away from the present.

In Chapter 8 I told part of what happened in a session with Gary, a Vietnam medic, when he came to see me unannounced and very upset after delivering a load of dried blood to a laminated wood products company. The smell had set off all kinds of memories and intrusive thoughts of Vietnam. He had to talk and was very agitated initially. This is the rest of the session:

Much of my time in Vietnam I was covered with dried blood. I hated the smell. Sometimes to get it off, I scrubbed so hard I made myself bleed. At the beginning I blamed the Vietnamese for everything. I hated them. In a dust-off we picked up a Vietnamese woman with a little child. The child was very ill and dehydrated. I had some pediatric catheters because sometimes I needed them when I couldn't start anything bigger on some of the wounded vets. I stuck the little girl seven times trying to get an IV started. The mother sat there impassively. I started to say to myself that she was sure a cold-hearted bitch. Then she started crying. Tears gushed forth. She cried a long time. By the end of that flight my hate had disappeared. The Vietnamese are human beings also.

Our dust-off base was a couple of miles from an ARVN [Army of the Republic of Vietnam] camp. We got a call to go there. Two deuce-and-a-halves [large army transport trucks] had hit anti-tank mines. Our chopper took off and came right down to them. From the air it looked like a giant had kicked over two Tonka Toys. There were two American advisors with the ARVNs. One of the Americans was evacuating his more seriously wounded comrade from the trucks. He carried him to the chopper. After I loaded his buddy, I helped him. I then realized to my surprise that he had been able to carry his buddy to the chopper even though he himself was missing his left arm above the elbow and his right foot at the ankle. Despite this he helped me with the other wounded. All he said was, "Gawd, it's awful." He was not bleeding at all. Shock was saving his life.

I saw shock save men and kill them. We were called to a new firebase. Some incredible idiot had set off the perimeter mines. They had been linked so that in a mass attack they could be set off altogether. Only problem was, many of the base personnel were out working on the perimeter when it was set off. Almost everyone was dead. One guy was alive and only lightly wounded in the legs – nothing that should have been life threatening. We put him on a stretcher and put in an IV. I could see him going into shock and starting to die right in front of me. I tried talking to keep him awake, but it wasn't working. Then I think I was inspired. I started swearing at him. I called him everything but a white man. I told him to just go ahead and die. I got out his wallet. There was a woman's picture there. I said we would rob him after he died and then find his wife and screw her. At this point he finally woke up and got so agitated we had to restrain him! I sometimes wonder if he ever figured out that what I did saved his life.

At this point we were both laughing almost uncontrollably. Thinking of having to threaten a man like that to reverse the effects of shock was just too funny. There is plenty of macabre humor in war, and I am convinced that being able to appreciate it has life-long benefits.

It also helps to be able to laugh at oneself. Guy (see Chapter 9) lost both legs and most of his right hand in Vietnam. A few years ago he was faced with rotator cuff surgery on his left shoulder, his only intact limb after the war. He found himself very anxious about the surgery and finally blurted out to his therapist, "If they screw up this surgery, I could be handicapped!" His therapist burst into laughter at the irony of this statement coming from someone missing two limbs already. Guy was able to laugh as well. Guy admits the laughter not only diminished his anxiety but also helped him begin exploring the emotional significance of some of his previous traumatic amputations.

Roger was a Marine Corps rifleman who spent 13 intense months in Vietnam. We have worked together for many years as I have helped him process his war experiences, and he has benefited from medication for hyper-alertness and insomnia. He lives on modest means and enjoys purchasing much of what he needs at garage sales. He likes to get there early before the crowds. He was recently leaving a garage sale with a purchase when he stepped on a Styrofoam packing "peanut" that was lying partially concealed in the grass. This piece of Styrofoam crunched underfoot in a way that to Roger's ears sounded just like stepping on a certain type of mine in Vietnam. He immediately froze with his foot pressing firmly down on the "peanut." Combat patrol protocol demanded that he hold that position until another Marine could come up and slip a knife under his boot. Then with the second Marine pressing down firmly with his bayonet, Roger would be able to lift his foot, get a large rock, and place it on the mine detonator. The second Marine would carefully remove his knife, and from a safe distance they would shoot the rock off the mine – causing it to detonate harmlessly.

Roger looked around, but there were no other Marines nearby! He could see several of the Styrofoam peanuts in the grass around him. Intellectually he knew he was at a garage sale and not in Vietnam and that he was standing on a piece of Styrofoam and not a mine, but all his combat instincts were screaming at him that he was one false move away from dismemberment or death. Finally he began to laugh at the absurdity of his predicament, and as he told the story we both began laughing in the session as well. His laughter freed him from his paralysis and he was able to walk away with his purchase.

Roger's experience – laughing at his own combat-conditioned response – is an archetypal healing response. Laughter is so much more effective at reversing this type of conditioning than getting angry. Anger often seems to reinforce the fear or threat-based conditioning, while laughter begins to dispel it, just as it did for Roger.

Doug, one of my Korean War vets, had gathered with his squad in a protected gully just after dawn to share some hot cocoa and relax during a lull in the fighting. A corporal from the company CP (command post) had brought up copies of the US Army newspaper, *Stars and Stripes*, which they were all reading. One of the articles described an unnamed regiment that was engaged in heavy combat on the front lines. One of the newer privates, referring to the article with a hint of awe in his voice said, "It sounds like them poor bastards in that outfit are sure catching hell!" Their squad leader looked at him in disbelief and growled, "You dumb ass, that's us they're talking about." The rest of the men could not contain their laughter, nor could the private. The vet telling the story gets pleasure out of that bit of humor to this day.

In a recent group discussion several of the vets fell into a mournful discussion of their failing health. Ray, a WWII vet, finally deadpanned, "I can't get much done anymore. I have the time to do a lot now that I am retired, but before I can get started I've wasted half the day hunting for my hearing aid, glasses, false teeth, and car keys." We laughed so hard we could hardly breathe. A dreary discussion of failing health was transformed into a lighthearted but meaningful exploration of the physical and emotional challenges of aging.

During another group discussion focusing on the recent reactivation of the men's war memories by current war news, one WWII vet, Jerry, quipped, "I forget the things I want to remember and remember the things I want to forget." This insightful bit of humor was followed by another

WWII vet, Ken, deadpanning, "The war news doesn't disturb my sleep much anymore, because by the time I go to bed I have forgotten what was said." The men's laughter at these two comments was much more therapeutic than feeling continued resentment about still being saddled with unpleasant and distressing war memories more than 50 years after their wars.

One of my WWII vets always ends each visit with at least one good joke. Last time he had two:

> I went to see my family physician this week. He asked me as he walked into the exam room, "Mr. K what seems to be the problem?" I was honest with him and said, "I *seem* to be aging." [Emphasis by the patient]

After I had finally stopped laughing, my patient continued:

> You know, Doc, we have talked many times about how important it is to forgive our enemies. Last Sunday our minister was preaching just on that topic. He pointed out how forgiving them can eventually turn them into friends. He asked the congregation if there was anyone who had no enemies. Way in the back one of the oldest members of our congregation finally raised her hand. Our minister asked her to come forward. When she was up front next to him he said, "Sister Margaret would you please share with us all how it is that you no longer have enemies." She turned and looked at us and then growled, "I outlived all them bastards!"

He shares his sense of humor with everyone who has the sense to listen. It always lightens my day.

Men can make a healthy joke out of the grimmest circumstances. Larry was leading a Special Forces team that ambushed a VC unit at night. They killed eleven armed combatants, one of whom turned out to be a woman carrying a small baby in a backpack. The baby needed immediate evacuation, as they were deep in the jungle with nothing to feed it. Dehydration was setting in, and its crying was endangering them all. At that time in Vietnam the American-piloted helicopters were only allowed to come for a dust-off if an American was wounded. Otherwise the South Vietnamese had to be called to do it. The Americans had been on stand-by and were much closer, so Larry's team went ahead and called them. They put blood and bloody bandages all over an unwounded man and put the baby in his arms. When the dust-off came, they loaded both and evacuated them to safety. They were all laughing and smiling at their cunning trickery for weeks, delighted that the little baby survived because of their ruse.

Sometimes humor gets to the truth in ways nothing else can. Fred, who fought in Korea and Vietnam, had taken a day off to go fishing with his seven-year-old grandson. According to Fred, and for no apparent reason the boy asked:

"Grandpa, do they fight wars at night?"
"Yes." There was a pause.
"Grandpa, do they fight wars on holidays?"
"Yes." There was a little longer pause.
"Grandpa, do they fight wars on Saturday and Sunday?"
"Yes."

The pause was even longer and Fred could see that his grandson was finding all this very hard to accept.

"Then Grandpa, why do they fight wars?!"

As Fred concludes the story, he and I are both smiling at this innocent child's disbelief about all those good holidays and weekends ruined by war. Fred admitted he could not come up with an explanation that seemed believable to his grandson about why men would waste so many good fishing days fighting wars.

Using humor is almost mandatory for both the vets and the staff. When we are all emotionally wrung out from intense discussions, I have learned from the vets to occasionally say, "Let's take a break. Each man has to share one of the funniest things that happened to him in the war." Their humor can be marvelously refreshing.

Note

1   *Reader's Digest* has a humor section "Laughter is the Best Medicine" but I don't think the phrase is original to them.

Chapter 12

Sleep and Medication

When I was a teenager we had dairy cows. That meant arising every day at 5 a.m. to milk them. Ever since I left the farm, I wake up each morning at 5 a.m., remember with gratitude that I don't have to milk the cows, and go back to sleep. I have been trained by all those years of getting up and milking cows to awaken at that time. It is simple but effective conditioning that continues to affect my behavior decades later.

The conditioning for combat vets is many times more intense and serious. For example, Ray, a Marine who served as a gunner on the aircraft carrier *Enterprise* in the Pacific, tells me that they would often spends days and even weeks at a time at "general quarters," meaning at their battle stations. They would sleep and eat there if they could:

> It was one of the reasons we never got sunk or knocked out of the war. Those new ships and crews would show up in the fleet, and the crews would be sunbathing – no one at battle stations. Before you knew it, they had taken a bomb hit or kamikaze and were ablaze and fighting for their lives. Our Captain was hard but he kept us alive.

This regimen programmed Ray to get very little sleep. Later in life, he was up and unable to sleep, so he would go out and farm in the middle of the night. He was farming in the dark when he had an accident that cost him his arm.

Combat infantrymen learn to sleep very lightly. If things are quiet they sleep four hours and then have four hours of guard duty. When things are quiet for the Navy, it is four hours on and four hours off. Sleep naturally comes in three to four hour cycles. What this means for many combat vets is that they will sleep three to four hours on a good night and no more.

War conditions men to be hyper-alert. Any little noise wakes an ex-combatant. And when a combat vet is roused he comes fully and completely awake, alert to any potential intruder or unusual activity. Adrenalin has been activated, and it can be very difficult to return to sleep.

In each four-hour sleep cycle, humans will have at least one cycle of intense dreaming. During this time the eyes move back and forth without opening; and a mechanism in the brain keeps the rest of the body motionless. This is the REM or rapid eye movement sleep stage. In young children the mechanism that keeps the body motionless during sleep is not fully developed, so little children move more and even sleepwalk while dreaming. This mechanism also seems to deteriorate as we age, so the elderly tend to move around more in their sleep, often waking themselves or their partners. Often combat vets appear to override the mechanism that keeps them motionless in sleep. They have intense battle dreams during REM sleep and cry out or move. Their wives report that it can be dangerous to sleep with them when they are having battle dreams. They complain of being hit and even choked while their partners are dreaming. Ed's wife (see Chapter 1) told me the following:

> When he came home from the war he had awful dreams. I tried once to wake him and got a black eye for my efforts. I was lucky that was all that happened. He was so sorry about it. I knew he couldn't help it though. I just had to learn to never touch him while he was asleep.

Adult humans typically need about eight hours of sleep a night. When sleep-deprived, which many combat vets routinely are, they start dreaming very soon after falling asleep. The vets' minds need to catch up on all the lost dreamtime. Unfortunately, vets are prone to having "battle dreams" which get the adrenalin flowing. They start moving and wake up again after just a few minutes. This can make it very difficult for them to get adequate rest.

Night is an uncomfortable time for many vets. In most wars from WWII to the present, American forces enjoyed air superiority. This meant that the enemy preferred to attack at night when American air power was less effective. This was true both on land and at sea. It also meant that enemy attacks on American airfields often occurred at night, so US Air Force personnel developed heightened autonomic nighttime responsiveness also.

Most vets with combat exposure come home and have battle dreams every night for years. Sometimes they are not aware that they are dreaming, but their families are, because they cry out, move, talk and even shed tears in their sleep.[1] Vets feel more vulnerable at night, so they often have a weapon nearby – under a pillow, on the nightstand, under the mattress – so they can quickly deal with any intruder. The only people who have any reason to fear vets are burglars. They should understand that they have a higher than usual likelihood of being shot as a misperceived enemy infiltrator if they break into a vet's home.

Being sleep deprived, combat vets often struggle with daytime drowsiness, poorer concentration and greater irritability. They often sleep better in the daytime than at night and can make good night shift employees. Most vets would sleep better if a reliable armed guard stood watch as they slept. That is the way it is supposed to be in combat, and their unconscious knows it.

Most of the vets I see have difficulty sleeping at least occasionally and request help for their insomnia. I prescribe a variety of medications for them. What helps any particular vet depends on the side effects he experiences, his response and his other symptoms. Often trazodone, benzodiazepines, low doses of antidepressants, and several other less commonly used meds can be effective; some reduce nightmares as well. Most men are helped by appropriate medications to some degree without annoying side effects or any long-term problems. They sleep better, concentrate better and are less irritable.

Occasionally the drugs can be too effective. Boyd was always complaining of not sleeping, and I tried many different meds with only modest success. Finally I tried an older med, nortriptyline. When I saw Boyd next he had the medicine bottle in hand, and giving it to me declared:

"I'll never take that again!"
"Why, what happened?"
"Anyone could have snuck up on me and done anything!"
"What do you mean?"
"I slept like a log; that was the problem. When I woke up, eight hours had passed and I had no idea! I was too deeply asleep. That just isn't right!"
"But Boyd, that was what we wanted, wasn't it?"
"Well, not like that. It just isn't safe!"

The bottom line was that Boyd didn't feel comfortable sleeping soundly. It disturbed him more than sleeping poorly. It was more important for a combat Marine like him to be able to respond quickly to any threat at night than it was to sleep deeply. We never used the medication that worked best again. He was not ready for it. This has happened to me with enough vets that I now discuss it with them before trying any sleep meds.

Sometimes a vet may appear to have a sleep problem that ends up being something quite different. Several years ago a Korean vet in his early 60s reluctantly came to see me. He was retired but active. He loved to fish and be in the outdoors. He was happily married. For the last year he had been sleeping much less, as well as having more nightmares and intrusive thoughts of the war. He found himself tired and irritable during the day. He admitted that this was how it was for several years after the war, but he had not had these symptoms for three decades before they reappeared.

While in Korea he had been severely wounded in the thigh during a Chinese attack. His unit's position had been overrun in the dark, and he and a close buddy had become separated from the unit. His buddy could have escaped but refused to leave without him. They hid in an old irrigation ditch and evaded the Chinese by lying low. Almost a day later, under cover of darkness, they managed to crawl back to their lines despite his painful wounds. His buddy's help kept the horror of that day from ending with his death or capture, but his wounds were serious enough that he was hospitalized for several months and never returned to combat.

I searched for a cause for his increased symptoms. I wondered if he had lost a family member recently. "No." Were there problems in his marriage? "No." Were troubling world events reminding him of his war experiences? "No." After exploring these and other possibilities, we were unable to identify any reason for his problem sleeping and the increase of symptoms. We went ahead with medication. He agreed to take a low dose of trazodone to help him sleep. A few weeks later in a follow-up session he was doing somewhat better. He was sleeping more and felt less irritable. Still, he had some nightmares and in the daytime continued to experience intrusive and troubling thoughts of the war. At this meeting he complained of considerable pain in his old wound. As we discussed this, he revealed that the pain had started becoming more noticeable about a year before and bothered him most at night. We agreed to increase the trazodone, but I also called one of our surgeons who agreed to fit him into his busy clinic in two weeks to look at his leg. I started him on ibuprofen 600mg three times a day to try to reduce the leg pain.

Two weeks later the surgeon called. He had X-rayed the leg and examined the patient. The shrapnel was all well encapsulated and no surgery was indicated. The patient had told him that the ibuprofen was working much better than the trazodone. The leg pain was better and he was sleeping great as long as he took the ibuprofen. He had stopped the trazodone, and the nightmares and intrusive thoughts were almost completely gone on the ibuprofen alone! He told the surgeon that the ibuprofen was a great sleep medication.

A few months later we met again. Things were just as the surgeon had told me. The symptoms were once again in full remission. My vet was sleeping well. It became apparent that his increased physical activity after his retirement had inflamed his old leg wound. This had bothered him mostly at night and caused him to involuntarily start thinking more about Korea. He had more nightmares and disturbed sleep. The leg also bothered him more in the day, generating the intrusive thoughts of the war. The whole process was reversed when we treated the leg pain with the ibuprofen. It took away the traumatic memory cue and solved the problem. The cure for his PTSD symptoms was ibuprofen for the inflammation and pain – not trazodone for the insomnia.

Being chronically sleep deprived can have a number of immediate and longer-term consequences. Sleep deprivation is one of the major factors that lead men to break down in combat. I believe it is more important than fear but probably less important than grief. Some of the psychiatrists in WWII recognized this and used this knowledge to treat acute cases of "combat fatigue." The standard treatment called for using high doses of phenobarbital or other soporifics to keep combatants asleep for 48–72 hours at a time.

In the case of the pilot described in Chapter 2 it was very effective. He got into trouble initially because he was having battle dreams every night and was sleeping only a few hours. Because of his sleep deprivation, he was taking a powerful stimulant to overcome his daytime drowsiness and maintain his alertness while flying. The stimulant, amphetamine, was actually exacerbating his tendency for flashbacks. In his case, he was seeing German fighter aircraft that were not there while he was flying his missions. We have learned since WWII that amphetamines can cause hallucinations. When the pilot was taken off flight duty, the deep narcotic-induced sleep and subsequent two weeks of rest resolved his acute symptoms enough to allow him to return to effective combat flying.[2]

Tim, the 1st Division medic who broke down from grief after one of the last of the original men in his company was killed (see Chapter 7), initially was treated with two days of sleep therapy, or narco-therapy as it was called then. When he awoke he was no longer uncontrollably crying, but unfortunately no other treatment was offered for his heart-rending grief. One reason he broke down in uncontrollable tears of grief was sleep deprivation, along with the sheer physical and mental fatigue of prolonged combat. Unfortunately it took over 40 years before his traumatic grief was effectively addressed.

The use of the phrases "combat fatigue" and "operational fatigue" arose in part because men often looked so exhausted when they broke down from acute battlefield PTSD. Under the powerful stimulus of combat, men can go up to two days without sleep and still reason and function. If they are forced to go beyond that, their functioning rapidly deteriorates and they become much more susceptible to breaking down.[3,4] The three main causes of wartime breakdown are traumatic grief, exhaustion and fear, in that order. All are usually present and seem to exacerbate each other, but grief and exhaustion are the dominant causes in most cases.

One essential function that occurs in sleep is the normalization of our blood pressure. I worry that a combat vet's sleeping blood pressure never returns to the low levels that occur in un-traumatized civilians. Now that we have instruments that can assess blood pressure while a person sleeps, we could study vets and get a better idea of the long-term effect of combat exposure on their blood pressure.

There is some evidence that chronic sleep deprivation predisposes individuals to anxiety attacks, depression and even more severe mood disorders. Given their symptoms of hyper-arousal and insomnia, one drug vets certainly do not need is caffeine. It arouses them further and adds to their difficulty sleeping. I tell them it is analogous to pouring gasoline on a fire. Some vets who are more hyper-aroused find that certain mood stabilizers and antidepressants decrease their arousal, treat their insomnia and improve their ability to deal more effectively with life. Combat vets can develop depression, panic disorder, schizophrenia and bipolar disorder just like anyone else. In that case they need all the appropriate medications used to treat those conditions effectively.

Effective use of medication to treat the hyper-arousal, irritability and insomnia that frequently plague combat vets often opens the door to the treatment of the more serious issues of traumatic grief and guilt that have gnawed silently at them for years. One reason vets avoid dealing with these deeper issues is that trying to do so often sparks memories and feelings associated with the war that initially exacerbate the physical symptoms of PTSD – making coping and functioning at least transiently more difficult. When the more superficial physical and mental symptoms of insomnia, hyper-arousal and irritability are controlled by medication, men feel safe enough to delve into the deeper recesses of their souls. The effective treatment of the outward symptoms of PTSD by medications, relaxation and behavioral techniques, and other therapies promotes a positive therapeutic relationship. This often leads men to hazard exploring their more serious concerns with these same therapists. Thus, the effective treatment of the conditioned physical and mental responses to war can ultimately lead to more profound healing from the moral and emotional pain of killing, grief, and fears about breaking the soldier's trust that are the deepest emotional and spiritual wounds of war.

Notes

1   Bradley op. cit. p. 259.
2   Hastings op. cit. pp. 301–7.
3   Patten, George S. Jr., *War as I Knew it*, pp. 191, 334–5.
4   Moore op. cit. pp. 192–3, 195.

Chapter 13

The "Antidote Experience" and Its Use in Therapy

In 1989 I had a clinical encounter that began to open my eyes to a therapeutic force I had never previously perceived or understood. I now call it the "antidote experience." This antidote event has the power to positively reshape a person's experience of war. Let me share with you that encounter in the words I used at the time:

> Our psychiatric evaluation office is across the hall from our audiology clinic. I had just finished seeing a walk-in patient when I heard loud voices outside the door. I opened it to find a veteran steaming mad, arguing with our audiologist. In an effort to defuse the situation I invited him in and asked what the problem was. He informed me he had just driven 300 miles to our VA from his home "to get a hearing aid." He was 68 years old, and he knew he had damaged his hearing in the Navy in WWII. He served on the battleship *North Carolina*. He made it clear he had never sought any VA services before. He had assumed that if he just drove over, he would be helped. Now, "can you believe it?" He was being told that he "wasn't eligible" for a hearing aid!
>
> I barely managed to suppress a smile about his naïvety. Given the arcane eligibility rules of the VA, there is almost nothing harder to be eligible for than a hearing aid. I went ahead and asked him when he first thought he might have suffered hearing damage in the service.
>
> "We were near the Solomon Islands. I was below deck on a work detail. Two torpedo hits knocked us all flat and I couldn't hear for a while. We started to evacuate and close off watertight doors to prevent further flooding. My best friend and I were the last to leave. He got his foot caught in the door. The seawater was pressing against it so hard we could not get his foot out. The water was rushing in around the seal. I grabbed a fire ax and tried to pry it back open. My buddy yelled, 'Cut it off' – meaning his leg. I knew he was right. Otherwise he would drown. I chopped his leg off below the knee. He was screaming. I carried him out of the compartment and dogged down the hatch. I put a tourniquet on and carried him to the pharmacist's mate."
>
> I was no longer smiling inside. After a pause I asked if there were any other experiences he wanted to share.
>
> "We were loading ammunition – powder cartridges. I was topside guiding the hoist. Six of my shipmates were in the magazine stowing the powder. Just after

I let down the first load there was an explosion that knocked me off the hoist onto the deck. I was unconscious briefly. When I came to I was bleeding from both ears. We immediately went into the magazine. The whole ship should have been destroyed. For some God-blessed reason only one powder cartridge had exploded. My mates were just pieces and red smears. We cleaned the mess up."

I did not know quite what to say, and there was another longer pause. I wondered why this man had never been to see us before. I finally asked, "How do you cope with these memories?"

"They never trouble me anymore. The war was one of the best experiences of my life."

I was stunned but tried not to show it. "What do you think about when you think about the war?"

For a moment he got a little teary-eyed.

"I always think about the bravest thing I ever saw."

Another pause. I asked, "What was the bravest thing you ever saw?"

"The war was almost over, but we didn't know it at the time. I was still on the *North Carolina*. I had advanced in rank and taken on a new rating. I was the talker between the bridge and our two Kingfisher spotter planes. We were about two miles off the coast shelling targets deep inland with our sixteen-inch guns. Our first spotter plane was hit by anti-aircraft fire and the pilot bailed out. He was floating in the water about two hundred yards from shore. He was being shot at; you could see the splashes around him. Our second Kingfisher was waiting on the catapult. The pilot requested permission to be catapulted off so he could land on his pontoons and try to rescue the downed pilot. Our five-inch guns were pounding anything on shore that was shooting at the downed pilot. The captain refused, saying it was pure suicide. The pilot persisted, begging to be given the chance to rescue the downed pilot before he was killed. Through the binoculars we couldn't tell if he was alive or dead. The captain took the microphone. He was yelling at our second Kingfisher pilot. Finally he said, 'All right, you can go. But as God is my judge, I will not take responsibility for your death also.'

"The Kingfisher catapulted off and landed next to the downed pilot. He was alive, and grabbed the pontoon. The second pilot began slowly taxiing back towards the ship, dragging the other pilot with him. We could see pieces of the plane falling off as it was hit by shellfire. Our five-inch guns kept pounding the shoreline. The plane arrived and was hoisted aboard. Both pilots were wounded but alive. The Kingfisher was so shot up we just dumped it over the side. I never think of the war without thinking of this event."

We were both quietly crying. I wrote the first two stories down in the chart just in case he ever applied for service-connected disability to obtain the hearing aids. He was no longer angry. I tried to explain all he would have to go through to become eligible for a hearing aid. He said it was getting late and he still had a long way to drive. He guessed he would just try to get a hearing aid on his own. I was reminded again of a comment one of my Vietnam vets once made to me. "War brings out the best and the worst in people." This was one time it seemed the best had overcome the worst.[1,2]

As time went on I thought a lot about this encounter. This man gave no indication that he was bothered in any way by his wartime experiences. The *North Carolina* was in the thick of naval combat in the South Pacific. Was it true that this one event always came to mind when he was thinking about the war? It was an act of love and bravery. Doug from the Chapter 10 would have quietly said, "Christ-like," and quoted John 15:13 from the Bible. Can being involved in an event like this actually override the hellish memories and usual negative impact of war?

I thought about another experience I had when I was in my last year of residency at Yale Medical School. I had written an article with the vice-chair of the department, Boris Astrachan, and we were on a panel in Detroit presenting it at the National Conference of Community Mental Health Centers. Another member of the panel was Jack Wilder, the vice-chair of the psychiatry department at Albert Einstein Medical School in New York. We finished early, and the three of us shared a taxi to the airport to try to get an earlier flight out. We were unsuccessful and now had a two-hour wait. Jack proposed a trip to the bar and said he would buy. Boris said that he would buy the second round, but they would have to find a bar that served fruit juice as well, since I was a "clean-living Idaho farm boy and never drank." Jack paused, looked at me intently, and with his eyes moistening wanted to know if I knew a man he served with in the 1st Marine Division on Guadalcanal. Of course I didn't, but Jack proceeded to tell me all about this other "clean-living Idaho farm boy."

They had been in the same platoon. All Jack could talk about was this man's singing. He said, "He was a church-going Mormon and he must have sung in the choir. When we were depressed and feeling hopeless, we would ask him to sing to us. He had a beautiful baritone voice and sang the most soothing hymns. When I think of Guadalcanal, I hear him singing."

At the time this had no significance to me. Later, when I learned more history and had treated three men who were there, it took on greater importance. You have to know that Guadalcanal was hell in 1942 for the Marines. They were dropped off with inadequate supplies to capture and hold an airfield the Japanese had nearly completed. During the seven months the Marines were there before being relieved, malaria and other jungle diseases afflicted almost everyone. Food and ammunition were inadequate and the fighting was merciless. Few thought they would survive.

After my encounter with the *North Carolina* seaman, I thought again of Jack and what he said of Guadalcanal and his hymn-singing buddy. I had interacted with him on several occasions and he was very relaxed and jovial – not my image of a Guadalcanal 1st Marine Division vet!

About that time I came across a passage in Primo Levi's autobiographical account of living through the horror of the Holocaust. He talks about the importance of his relationship with a guard named Lorenzo:

> However little sense there may be in trying to specify why I, rather than thousands of others, managed to survive the test, I believe that it is really due to Lorenzo that I am alive today; not so much for his material aid, as for his having constantly reminded me by his presence, by his natural and plain manner of being good, that there still existed a just world outside our own, something and someone still pure and whole, not corrupt, not savage, extraneous to hatred and terror; something difficult to define, a remote possibility of good, but for which it was worth surviving ... The personages in these pages are not men. Their humanity is buried, or they themselves have buried it, under an offence received or inflicted on someone else. The evil and insane SS men, the Kapos, the politicals, the criminals, ... But Lorenzo was a man; his humanity was pure and uncontaminated, he was outside this world of negation. Thanks to Lorenzo, I managed not to forget that I myself was a man.[3]

I knew this concept could be important to my work, but I still didn't grasp how to use it. Levi seemed to be saying that the example of one good man had kept him alive through Auschwitz – had helped him maintain his "humanity" when everyone around seemed to have lost theirs. Can one remarkable "good" be an effective antidote for so much evil? What was remarkable about Lorenzo, according to Levi, was nothing obviously heroic, but instead, his simple and consistent kindness to all around him, while everyone else was cold and brutal.

Ken (mentioned first in Chapter 3), a mortarman in the 84th Infantry Division and a member of my first WWII PTSD group, gave me a book written about another company in the 84th. It was part of his effort to broaden my education. He told me, "This book tells it like it really was." For Ken that was saying a lot. He could attend many group sessions and never say a word. I took him seriously and read it.

Ken was right. Written by the company's surviving officers and men, *The Men of Company K* comes as close to being there as a book can. The men met regularly for reunions and finally decided to tell what their war was like before they all died. Among other things, the book and their writing process illustrate the natural therapeutic power of reunions and writing honestly about one's experiences.

One incident captured my attention. For a few weeks the unit was opposite the Germans in a brief stalemate with entrenched lines at the Roer River. They had a good medic named Mellon, also referred to as "Doc Mellon" or just "Doc." The authors describe an incident involving Mellon:

> Several men had reported hearing a GI yelling for help during the night. At daybreak they finally spotted him lying helpless near the riverbank. Battalion told us a patrol from a cavalry unit had lost a man, and we decided to send out a stretcher team at nightfall to rescue him.
>
> Mellon thought the man needed help right away. He didn't check with the company officers; he knew they would veto his rescue scheme. Pulling on his Red Cross bib, Doc stood in the open to make sure the Germans spotted him. He then walked slowly toward the river. He worked his way through a roll of concertina wire and crossed a small creek. Mellon reached the wounded man and found he was shot through the ankle; the bones were shattered. The fellow was conscious, but suffering from shock and unable to move. Realizing he would be unable to carry his patient a quarter mile to the safety of our positions, Doc bandaged the wound, squeezed a morphine syrette into the man's side, and returned slowly to the company area.
>
> Doc remembered seeing a vehicle in a ruined shed that might solve his problem. He looked it over and headed again for the river. "It was an old beat-up wheelbarrow with a wooden body, no sides, and with a metal-rimmed wheel. It was heavy and bulky, and I had one hell of a time getting it through the concertina wire." Doc ripped his hands on the wire, but finally wrestled his wheelbarrow over the obstacle and through the creek. He checked the wounded man's bandage and loaded him on the wheelbarrow.
>
> By that time the word had spread up and down the line, and every man in K Company was watching apprehensively. Men yelled across the river to the Germans, "Okay, hold it, hold it," and the Germans hollered back, "Okay," but when Doc began his trip toward safety, one German fired. It was impossible to tell if the shot was aimed at Doc, but word was passed not to return fire. The worst that could happen was for Doc and his patient to be caught in a crossfire.[4]

Here we have an incident of the highest drama and potential impact on the psyches of the men of Company K. All are watching and wound up to a high emotional pitch. If the Germans kill Doc, the spirit of revenge and retaliation will reap a bitter and savage harvest in the feelings and subsequent actions of these men. But what if Doc's heroism and self-sacrifice are rewarded by German restraint and mercy? Either for good or ill this could be one of the most memorable and influential events of the war for all involved. The authors continue:

> The rescue proceeded in agonizingly slow motion. Balancing the man on the wheelbarrow, Doc pushed it slowly across the muddy ground to the little creek. He stopped, carried the man across on his shoulder, set him down, and went back for the wheelbarrow. To get through the belt of concertina wire, Mellon repeated the process.
>
> "All the way back," Doc remembers, "some crazy German bastard kept shooting at us. It was rifle fire, and some of it was mighty close. I told the guy to try and hold on, but he kept falling off the wheelbarrow and I'd have to lift him back on. He was hurting pretty bad. I'd swear at him and tell him to hold on tighter."
>
> When Doc and his cargo were within a 100 yards of safety, a German machine gunner opened fire, digging up spurts of mud only a few feet from the pair, but Doc plodded along deliberately, making no effort to hurry or take cover. As he finally pushed the wheelbarrow into an alley behind a ruined house at the edge of Linnich, a cheer went up from every man in K Company.
>
> After his patient had been evacuated to battalion aid, Doc came to the CP. Soaked to the crotch, covered with mud, one hand bandaged, Doc pulled out a cigarette and took a deep drag. "That settles it," he announced. "I've just decided. No more house calls." Had the Germans been trying to hit Doc? We had no way to know, but a protocol of sorts had been established between K Company and the German infantrymen on the opposite bank of the river. Several times during our weeks at Lindern, German aidmen had picked up casualties between the lines and we made it clear to our replacements that nobody was to interfere with such rescue efforts.[5]

I pondered the possible repercussions of witnessing such an event. I linked this incident involving "Doc Mellon" with Jack Wilder's singing Idaho farm boy in the hell of Guadalcanal. I saw a connection to the seaman on the *North Carolina* who watched the Kingfisher pilot demand the opportunity from his captain to submit himself to a hail of lead on the outside possibility that he might save a comrade in arms. And what about Primo Levi's attributing his survival of Auschwitz to the decent, human example of one man, Lorenzo? Was it possible that many men have antidote experiences that outweigh the poisonous horror of war? Are there thousands of combat vets out there who never need help because they participated in similar events, and these uplifting episodes of courage, self-sacrifice and mercy are what they remember above all else?

I returned the book to Ken and mentioned the incident involving "Doc Mellon." He knew about it but didn't witness it. He then said as his eyes lit up, "Our medic was the bravest man I ever saw." And then with deep sadness, "A lot of the very best ones like him got killed. He always went to where the men needed him most." A short time later he brought me a dog-eared newspaper article about his medic, written before he was killed. The article's author was Pvt. Arnold Ehrlich, but Ken could not remember what publication he cut it from, though he thinks it was *Stars and Stripes*:

Sgt. Robert E. Ward, of Princeville, Illinois, is much more than a brave man. He is a man who, according to the second battalion chaplain, Capt. John A. Morrison, "lives with a broken heart. He's had too many men die in his arms."

... At Gereonsweiler Ward, besides tending the sick and wounded of his own company, [he] evacuated at least 50 men from the entire regiment. The medic braved enemy fire from the front lines to return to the rear, collected six jeeps and one armored "weasel," supervising the evacuation through the entire night.

Again on January 8, Ward "covered the entire battalion front" in the Marcouray-Cielle sector, "personally attending and carrying to safety many wounded, constantly exposed to enemy fire, braving the hazards of mountainous terrain."

When there was hot fighting west of Devantave, Ward went to a draw to administer first aid to several wounded. Using two dead bodies as a shield against constant machine gun fire, the medic stayed in the dangerous spot for 10 minutes.

He soon left this position to go to the aid of First Battalion doughs pounded by mortar fire. An intense mortar barrage was in progress. Crossing an open hill under heavy machine gun fire, he continued to bring comfort to the wounded. After dark Ward organized stretcher parties, improvised makeshift stretchers, and continued to give medical attention for eight hours, evacuating at least 30 men.

Again at Cielle, still under relentless artillery and mortar fire, the first-aid man administered aid to and evacuated at least 23 wounded soldiers.

He is credited with "saving at least 100 lives."

... His company commander, Lt. D.E. Lawrence, of Spokane, Washington, speaks warmly of his courage and bravery in battle: "Ward's presence on the battle-ground is a high morale factor. He gives the boys confidence in the medics as a whole. He has been offered easier work at a higher rating but has refused. He says he can do more in the field."

... The second battalion executive officer, Maj. James Johnston, of Portland, Oregon, pays him a rare tribute: "Ward has been under more enemy fire than any other man in the battalion. In every battle we've been in Ward has been within yards of enemy fire. He has demonstrated more personal bravery than any man I've seen in combat. It is a great honor to recommend this man for the Distinguished Service Cross."

There was sadness in Ken for Ward's death, but it was very clear that Ward's actions and example meant a great deal to him, and his memory was a source of strength. "He even worked on us while he was wounded. It hurt me deep when he was killed."

I started exploring this with the men in group and began bringing it up with individual vets I was seeing. I think of it as fishing for healing and uplifting memories to balance the destructive ones. I began finding antidote experiences in almost everyone, and I wondered how I could have missed this therapeutic resource for so many years. I learned that if I want to foster the soldiers' moral recovery, it is every bit as important to explore these positive events in depth as it is the various forms of killing they experienced.

The Kingfisher pilot, the singing farm boy, Lorenzo, "Doc," and Ward displayed remarkable qualities, but they were not uncommon ones. On exploration, almost every vet saw similar acts of courage and self-sacrifice, and although sometimes reluctant to reveal it, many did something similar themselves. Two of my 8th Air Force vets, who were shot down and became POWs, mourn and honor the memory of their pilots. Why? On both occasions the pilots tried to hold their heavily damaged bombers steady enough for the crew to safely bail out. But what of the pilots? How did they leave? They had no ejection seats. They had no quick escape. When they left the controls, the heavily damaged planes' violent motion may have kept them from making any exit. I am sure that given their experience, the pilots knew that staying at the controls and allowing others to escape reduced their own chances of survival.

I discovered from some of my patients that each WWII aircraft carrier had armorers who risked their lives every day in the simplest, grimmest fashion to save the ship. Planes would return to the carrier with armed bombs that would not dislodge because the release mechanism had failed.[6] When the arresting gear hooked on landing, the plane's violent stop occasionally dislodged the armed bombs. The bombs had fuses at each end. They were designed not to explode until they had travelled a certain distance and had been released a certain amount of time, in order to ensure they never blew up the plane that dropped them. Two men were always waiting on deck. They would sprint to the rolling bombs and grab them like cowboys taking down a calf for branding. Each man would disarm an end of the bomb. By the time they reached the bomb, they only had seconds to do this. Can you imagine the courage to do this over and over? When I asked the sea-going Marine who first told me about this how it made him feel, he responded with tears in his eyes, "You couldn't believe their bravery. But it was their job and they did it all the time. You get used to that kind of bravery in war."

Once I bring it up, men can spend whole sessions talking about the acts of courage and self-sacrifice they witnessed. One of my Vietnam Special Forces vets thinks some helicopter pilots are the bravest of heroes. He speaks reverently of the man who flew in to rescue them after being ordered away:

> We were surrounded. The enemy had heavy weapons covering us. I thought having the chopper come in would just add to the death toll. He came in anyway, and though most of us got wounded, we all got out. How do you thank a man for that? All of our children exist because of him.

How do I now use this antidote experience principle in therapy? The first step is to find the story. Where I go from there depends on the story and the man involved. It is a rich process of discovery. The answers and uses are uniquely individual.

Here is one example. In a recent group therapy session one of those "hero pilots," Fred, began exploring some of the moral pain of his war. "I cannot get the image of that child out of my head." He had just helped capture a Vietcong-controlled village. White phosphorus had been dropped to drive the VC out, followed by a helicopter-borne infantry assault. He helped bring in the infantry. When the fighting was done, a woman from the village brought her infant and handed it to him. The dead child had holes burnt clear through it by the phosphorus:

> It is my worst memory of the war. When white phosphorus lands on someone, it can eat a hole right through them. I didn't drop the phosphorus, but I was certainly part of the team that did. We killed that child. I could understand and share her pain. I had two children back home.

He wondered where he would start if he wanted to "be right before God" for all the things he participated in while at war in Korea and Vietnam:

> There are so many. In Korea the Chinese ambushed one of our ambulances. When I found them, the four medics had their heads cut off and their genitals in their mouths. It took a lot of killing over the next few weeks to get that rage out of me. You want to do more than kill the enemy, you want to smash them and rip them apart. But when you finish, it's not a good feeling. It weighs on you.

As the group session continued, Fred admitted that earlier that week a man
he had never met called his home and left a message:

> He wanted me to know that he and his squad were sharpening their bayonets
> because that was all they had to use against the North Vietnamese. When he
> heard our chopper coming in, it meant hope and ammo. He heard us do it many
> times that day and knew we took heavy fire each time. He just wanted me to
> know that the son he never would have had, except for our relief flights, had a
> child, and that he was now a grandpa.

This is the start. It begins with getting the positive out as well as the whole
truth about the negative. When asked, he admits that he never expected to
live through any of the relief flights that day.

> "Then why did you do it?" I asked.
> "You can't break the soldier's trust. That whole unit would have died if I
> didn't go in. I guess my men went with me because they weren't going to let
> me do it alone. I couldn't do it alone anyway. It was our job to help those
> surrounded on the ground. To do less was unthinkable to me. We weren't
> heroes. We were just doing our job."
> "If you hadn't gone in, how many would have died?"
> "It was a battalion trapped – maybe even hundreds."

I don't know how many lives saved make up for one killed. Can life and
death be measured that way? If you kill, does it matter that you also risked
your life and saved others? I do not understand the cosmic weights and
balances of justice and mercy. But I am willing to discuss it, and that day
in group the men did. Fred concluded by noting, "I believe in God. It is a
deep personal thing for me. All I ask for from my God is mercy. I don't
think he can forgive me for all I've done, but maybe he can be lenient."

Although nothing was fully resolved that day in therapy and probably
never will be, the discussion itself was necessary and helpful. We have
come back to it many times in our group sessions. Each time we explore it
a little deeper. The medic Ward was described in the news article as having
saved a hundred men. Yet the same writer said Ward "lives with a broken
heart." The antidote experiences I eventually hear from my vets don't
resolve all the moral and emotional pain. But as the poet from Chapter 10
said, they can add to "... a weights and measures system of stability and
growth, a way to move on ..." They do provide a therapeutic balance to the
worst of the memories. The key for the therapist is to look for them and
then use them appropriately.

I have learned that the therapist can sometimes be successful in getting new antidote experiences to occur. Think of Boyd getting together with Guy (see Chapter 9). Boyd thought that clamping the arteries in Guy's stump to keep him alive had probably condemned Guy to a life of depression and misery without his legs. That is a typical thought for a young healthy male who believes that becoming physically disabled is worse than death. At that age he does not have the experience and wisdom to appreciate the incredible ability of the human spirit to overcome physical and emotional challenges and make happiness out of hell. Later, when he thinks about that wartime experience, he is still applying his youthful frame of reference to it. Boyd's therapist knew there was a high likelihood Guy was alive and had overcome his physical limitations to the degree that he had found reasonable happiness and meaning for himself. She saw nothing to be lost and potentially much to be gained in trying to get the two men together. She was right. It became a great healing antidote experience.

The same happened, but even more so, to Roland (see Chapter 9) when he met the Captain he was sure he had not saved. He discovered that his Captain had not only lived, but lived well.

Both reunions and group therapy have the potential to create new antidote experiences that allow a more mature and positive interpretation and reframing of past war traumas. In reunions it occurs through reprocessing events with the actual participants. In group therapy it occurs by reprocessing with other trusted, knowledgeable combatants. In both cases the therapist can facilitate healing by encouraging the sharing and exploration of meaningful experiences and emotions among all involved. This can happen only when therapy has advanced to the point that the vets are ready to face their worst fears honestly.

Finally, my veterans have provided me with a chest full of valuable healing stories that I can draw on to help other vets. I can use these stories to help them see their experiences in a more positive light. The story of one man's experience can become an antidote for another man's pain. The impact of sharing therapeutic stories is not always predictable, but when done selectively it is usually helpful. I have never seen it be harmful.

For example, after treating both Ed and Frank for a period of time (see Chapter 1), I shared with each the other's experience of killing or not killing an American comrade dying from untreatable wounds. Ed had mercifully suffocated a man who begged Ed to put him out of his misery. Frank had declined to do such an act, but had sat with his three comrades to the end, providing them all the comfort he could. Both blamed themselves, Ed for mercifully killing and Frank for not "being man enough" to mercifully kill his wounded and dying comrades.

Ed's response to hearing about Frank's self-castigation for not having mercifully killed was sympathetic but low key. It did not have much appreciable impact on him. On the other hand, when Frank heard the details of what happened to Ed, he responded immediately. He felt freed from a dreadful burden. He could see that he would have blamed himself just as much if he had killed the three men as they requested as he had been blaming himself since then for not having killed them. Perceiving now that he had faced a "no win" situation, he could more readily forgive the young man he was then for actions taken in a situation that allowed no guilt-free or "correct" choice. He worked on this a few more sessions and left therapy much relieved. I ran into him casually a few years later and he said he had continued to process it and was no longer troubled by his actions.

Fourteen years have passed since 1989, and I still do not know how many combatants are like the sailor described in this chapter's first story or like Jack Wilder. When thinking of their war, these two remember above all else a pilot's act of inspiring bravery and sacrifice and a hymn-singing farm boy. I continue to wonder why focusing on these antidote experiences has such healing potential for some men. In some cases it is as if these experiences and memories prevented the veteran from developing long-lasting symptoms of PTSD. Some of the cases, like those of Lorenzo and the Idaho farm boy, are examples of humanizing a hellish situation. They spawn hope of a better world that might eventually prevail over the inhuman present. Other cases, like the medics' self-sacrifice and bravery, the armorers risking their all for their shipmates, and pilots flying through intense enemy fire to rescue and bring relief are examples of timeless, loving heroism. These men were transcendent upholders of "the soldiers' trust." They are examples of love prevailing over death and hell. If these displays of decent humanity and self-sacrifice are what a man remembers most from the war, how could his war experience cast any long-term shadow over his life?

I know in the VA we see only a small portion of those who experienced combat. I frequently encounter vets in other settings who I am convinced would benefit from some form of treatment. I invite them to come, but many do not. The vets I have in treatment often talk of vets they know who need treatment. Some they are able to persuade to come, but many do not. Many others appear untroubled by their experiences. I believe those who are less troubled have often made effective use of the healing forces described in this chapter and the last section of this book.

There are many more healing forces in addition to reunions, processing the war through writing, and antidote experiences that veterans make use of over the course of their lives that are not part of our traditional treatments. These healing forces – including spiritual conversions, healthy love relationships, meaningful service, and others – can be more effective than anything we offer in conventional psychiatric practice. My vets have enhanced my appreciation of many of these forces, and we will explore some of the more important ones in these final chapters.

Notes

1 Heiferman op. cit. Table of Contents, picture of *North Carolina*.
2 Goldstein, Donald M., Katherine V. Dillon and J. Michael Wenger, *The Way It Was, Pearl Harbor: The Original Photographs*, p. 21, picture of Kingfisher.
3 Levi, Primo, *Survival in Auschwitz*, p. 111.
4 Leinbaugh, p. 225.
5 Ibid p. 226.
6 Lopez op. cit. pp. 208–10.

Part III

The Hope of Redemption

This section of the book explores words and concepts of deep power, which often convey important variances of meaning for different individuals and cultures: sin, confession, mercy, forgiveness, redemption and love. I try to present, not what these concepts mean to me, but what they mean to the vets I treat and how they have used them to further their own recovery from war's grief and moral pain. I recognize that it is impossible for me to do this without my own values coming through to some degree. Nonetheless, I have tried the best I can to illustrate these principles through the lives of the men I have treated, as well as in the stories of combatants in similar circumstances. The men I have treated have reviewed what I have written about them in great detail. In many cases we have spent hours going over what I have said so their stories accurately reflect their words and thoughts and not my own. Nonetheless, I am presenting here what they taught *me*; so ultimately the conclusions about what their stories mean are mine.

I have struggled with my use of the word redemption. I have tried to use words like recovery or healing instead but they don't express fully what my patients have experienced and expressed to me. They feel that they have been plunged into hell by their war experiences and through powerful and miraculous healing forces can now live life again without overwhelming anger, bitterness and guilt. They can once again experience joy in life. Somehow the word redemption expresses their escape from hell into a renewed life better than any other single word.

Each man begins healing by having the courage to face the truth about himself and taking responsibility for his own recovery. This often leads to a change in perspective about himself and his war. This change of perspective can lead to developing mercy, taking reparative action, and giving and seeking forgiveness. Men speak of spiritual powers guiding and sustaining them. They use words like reconciliation, peace and redemption. They talk of loving relationships bringing meaning and purpose. They share their deepest feelings as they strive to overcome the hellish burden of war in their lives and find happiness and peace. If they can hope to recover from the emotional and spiritual wounds of war, can't we all have the same hope of recovery from our personal trauma and pain?

Chapter 14

Having the Courage to Face the Truth and Being Willing to Take Corrective Action

Many ex-combatants are trapped by fear. It is not fear of war or death. It is fear of facing the meaning of their past actions. They can be hounded by self-blame and guilt. My patients have taught me that running from their feared memories is never successful. Richard Clewell, a VA chaplain, touched powerfully on this in an article he wrote on the moral dimensions of the treatment of combat veterans. He talks about the killing expected of combatants and its impact on their views about themselves and then discusses briefly their unsuccessful attempts to forget what they have done:

> Often these combatants appear stuck in bad faith because of the irrevocable consequences of their actions, which resulted in concrete suffering or death. Trying to forget or outlive the events reinforces the feeling of bad faith and of breaking a covenant not only with others or with God, but also with one's own nature.[1]

Many vets do try to "forget or outlive" their war experiences. Sometimes they describe it as "running from them." I have heard so many times the refrain, "I have done everything I can to forget, but it has not worked. It only seems to get worse." The three types of experiences they are most commonly running from involve "breaking the Geneva Convention of the soul" (civilian casualties, killing of fellow soldiers, killing with deep hatred or elation, or battlefield justice), "breaking the soldier's trust" (feeling that in some way they let down their fellow combatants), and the killing of the humanized enemy. They often see these actions as irreparable moral transgressions and feel they are unforgivable. They feel estranged from God and humanity whenever they remember what they have done. Often when they finally turn and face their fears honestly, they discover that those fears are not as dreadful when faced in their full adulthood as they were when first encountered as teenage warriors.

One of the most destructive ways veterans run from their experiences is by turning to alcohol or, less commonly, drug abuse. Many vets begin using alcohol to lessen their insomnia and battle dreams. This can be transiently helpful, but when used chronically can lead to dependence and addiction. Alcohol disrupts the normal sleep patterns and architecture. Thus its long-term use actually exacerbates insomnia. When a man says, "Doc, I can't sleep without it," I know he is physically addicted and needs treatment. The alcohol also predisposes individuals to depression and anxiety disorders.

Alcohol abuse is common in combat vets. They have often been socialized into drinking while in the military. Free beer was not uncommon, and in some battle zones was easier to get than clean water. We have good data that the increased mortality seen in combat vets the first one to two years after the end of any war is attributable primarily to accidents. The accidents are often caused by increased alcohol abuse, although drug abuse and increased risk-taking may also be involved.[2,3] As mentioned previously, several years ago I took a survey of the 25 vets I then had in my two PTSD groups. Twenty had struggled with alcohol abuse after their combat time. All had finally given it up to enable them to move on more positively in life. The story of the D-Day medic Tim (Chapter 7), who needed alcohol treatment before getting his PTSD treated, is typical in this regard. He tried hard to bury his war experiences. He turned to alcohol as a way to numb his feelings and to try to sleep and forget.

Luther drove a tank and saw rough combat in France and Germany. He was captured in January 1945 in a German counterattack during the fighting at Herrlisheim.[4] He was atop his Sherman tank when he was shot through the helmet by a German sniper who had been hiding behind a white flag in a fake surrender. He sustained only a scalp wound and concussion and believes to this day that God changed the course of the bullet enough to spare his life. His unit was surrounded and forced to surrender, with almost every tank destroyed and most of the officers either killed or wounded. During his combat experience he saw many men he knew and loved burn to death in their tanks after they were hit by German cannon fire.

Although he was a POW only four months, Luther lost a great deal of weight and suffered severe frostbite. He was in a group of POWs stuffed into boxcars for transport to a POW camp. As the trip began, US planes strafed the boxcars – not knowing they were full of Americans. The train was destroyed, so the POWs were marched several hundred miles through Germany in the dead of winter to a POW camp in Austria. Luther was there when the war ended. During his time as a POW he suffered from starvation and lack of adequate clothing. In a picture taken at his liberation, he looked like a scarecrow.

After the war Luther was troubled by his war experiences and lost himself in booze. His wife and family left him, and he lived out of his camper as he wandered aimlessly for years. He finally "found God and redemption," got sober and remarried. He started writing poetry as part of his recovery, and that was when he sought treatment with the VA. In one poem he wrote eloquently of his time in combat and in another of his alcoholism. I have juxtaposed them because in my mind they are different sides of the same coin, and in Luther's life the ideas and feelings expressed were inextricably linked.

The Warrior

Through Hell I have wandered
I still see the flame,
And I'll swear before God
I'll never be the same.

For the peace that comes with death
Often I have yearned,
For I stood by helpless
As I watched my friends burn.
I still see them dying
I still hear their screams
As death claimed their bodies
And ended their dreams.

They say it's now over
That it's all in the past,
But it will never be ended
As long as memory will last.

Would anyone listen
If this story I should tell,
Of the time that I spent
Going through hell?

The Man from Another World

It's a world of another people
where the lonely wino lives.
Where they have no one to love them
for they have no love to give.
They've been robbed of all their pride
so they walk the streets in shame
in a world of another people,
just men without a name.
But if you watch them closely
sometimes a smile will cross their
    face.
Then you will know that they are
    thinking of some loved one
in that other world someplace.
Perhaps it's a son or daughter
they haven't seen in many years
but then, they take another drink
and wipe away the tears.
Yes, it's a world of another people
where you can never have a friend
but they keep walking down life's
    highway
till they come to the bitter end.

In the poem "The Warrior" you see Luther's pain over helplessly watching his beloved comrades burn. This is more than just witnessing a horrible death. These are men he trusted and loved and who felt the same way toward him. Why should he be alive and they dead? At a certain level he felt responsible for them. He could not escape from the fear that he had broken their trust. Somehow, he "should have" rescued them after their tanks were hit. It is analogous to the story of Herb (Chapter 6), who was unable to keep his solemn vow to his ball turret gunner to get him out, no matter what, if the plane was going down.

Both Herb and Luther, at a certain level, felt responsible for their comrades' deaths. They had committed one of the combatant's worst sins; they felt they had broken the soldier's trust. Each man feared talking, dreaming and thinking about it. In addition, Luther carried an added burden: "I know I killed children as we fought the Germans in France from village to town. I saw their little bodies mangled by my shells." Luther turned to drink as a way of forgetting. Herb just refused to talk about it. Both believed, "Talking about it will only make it worse." Both were running from something they had to face.

For a time Luther lost himself in the "other world" of the wino. There are many forms of alcoholism. This is only the most obvious. Many combat vets think their drinking is not a problem because they still have a job and family. They only drink to sleep. But they are still running from the war, and the continued drinking eventually jeopardizes their work and family life.

One of my vets says his daily marijuana "helps him cope." He is still avoiding truths he needs to face. The chronic marijuana use makes it seem less urgent to face those truths. It keeps him stuck in the same place in life for as long as he uses. "I'll start tomorrow" is the by-word of marijuana users, and 20 years later, if they are still using, "tomorrow" has never come.

The alcohol and drug abuse itself usually adds more shame and pain to these veterans' lives, leaving them with even more actions and events they want to forget. Unless they begin facing their fears and shame, their lives spiral down into further misery. In this state they often blame others for what has happened. It is just too searing to look deeply at one's self and one's own actions.

Many vets report that in this miserable condition the thing that made the most difference was having a friend or family member who stood by them and never gave up on them entirely, or who in desperation finally confronted them bluntly. Often the vets offered desperate prayers that they feel were answered – engendering renewed hope and courage. Many found further help in an organized religion or other spiritual traditions.

One combat vet told me of the miracle he experienced the fifth time he had been incarcerated for his drinking. He knew he had no power in his life anymore. Alcohol ruled all. He had prayed for help many times and had vowed never to drink again. Each time to his shame he had broken his vow. This time his prayer was even more desperate, and he acknowledged to God and himself that if God didn't help him, he could never stop. He felt a strong spiritual force touch his heart. When he left jail he had lost the desire to drink and hasn't done so since. Many men, who now look back on decades of sobriety, have told me similar stories. They describe their change in various ways but often use the phrase "through the grace of God" to describe how their "life," "heart," or "feelings" were changed. Some report, "I felt a spiritual force give me the special strength I needed to stop."

Alcoholics Anonymous (AA) has been the beginning of facing the truth for many of my vets. Step 4 of the 12 Steps of AA reads, "Made a searching and fearless moral inventory of ourselves." Step 5 reads, "Admitted to God, to ourselves, and to another human being the exact nature of our wrongs." Step 8 reads, "Made a list of all persons we had harmed, and became willing to make amends to them all." They start by applying these principles to the damage and misery that come from drinking. They end up using these same principles to begin the process of healing from the emotional and spiritual wounds of war.

A classic example is the story of Boyd. We discussed him earlier in Chapters 4 and 9. He left Vietnam having been decorated for his wounds and his gallantry, but saddled with two haunting demons. He had desecrated and mocked the corpse of a Vietcong he had killed. And he had broken the soldier's trust by saving a man's life only to "condemn him to a life of useless misery with no legs and only half a right hand."

Boyd came home and tried to pick up his life. He was soon drinking to sleep, forget and numb his feelings. He eventually became addicted to alcohol. His inability to face his demons and his continued drinking destroyed his first marriage. He remarried, struggling with alcohol the whole time. Love for wife and children motivated him to seek treatment. Supportive treatment and involvement in the cleansing principles of Native American "sweats" finally got him sober. Further treatment, spiritual work and courage led him to contact the Vietnamese and US governments to try to provide details so that the body of a Vietcong warrior could be properly recovered, returned to his family and honored. He began inviting other combatants to come to his "sweats" and participate in that purifying religious ceremony. Finally, he tried to contact the man he had "condemned to a life of useless misery," potentially face that man's bitterness, and humbly ask for forgiveness.

Facing his twin demons worked out very differently than Boyd anticipated. Neither government has shown any interest to date in Boyd's information about the location of this missing-in-action Vietcong. He keeps trying. Guy, when found, was not bitter, but loving, and greeted Boyd with joy as his lifesaver.

I treated Boyd for more than a decade. I gave him a little medication, encouraged him to get and stay sober, and tried to listen and understand. He will say to anyone who asks that it was helpful to see me. But I watched what happened. What started the deeper healing process was his beloved wife, who threatened to throw him out if he didn't get sober and accept treatment for his war trauma. She told him at the time, "I love you, but I can't deal with the enemy you carry within." His healing continued with his involvement with Native American spiritual traditions which helped him get and stay sober and begin facing his worst fears. And it was furthered by support from another VA therapist who helped him take concrete, redemptive action and face Guy's possible bitterness.

Part of facing the truth is recognizing that you are responsible for your treatment and recovery. It also requires you to look deeply at your own feelings and actions – sometimes with the help of a therapist. No one else can do it for you. One cowboy and hunting guide I treat said, "I had to stop hating and blaming others. I learned that hate and anger destroy the soul and keep you stuck where you are." He also had to overcome alcohol and marijuana abuse before facing his war trauma. Now he describes his struggle with his war memories and experiences this way: "You have to face them and work on them. If you don't, the dark ghost of the past creeps in and steals the present."

Wayne served as a rifleman in a LRRP (long range reconnaissance patrol) unit. He was involved in intense, deadly combat throughout his time in Vietnam. There were ambushes and prisoner snatches, killing the enemy face to face, and worries and grief about the deaths of close comrades. I have been involved in his treatment for 12 years. Wayne's treatment has followed a pattern similar to that of many combat vets. Speaking of his therapy he explains:

I think anyone who chooses therapy is choosing life over death, but unless one is desperate and can admit that, there may not be incentive or strength enough to try finding those little patches of light. After eleven years in the system, I look back on those first five years and think now that my greatest comfort during that time was learning I was not alone. The fellowship of vets from WWII, Korea, and Vietnam helped me find the strength to continue. This allowed me eventually to find a therapist [one of our social workers] who enabled me to connect the dots in my life and rediscover my feelings – to feel human again and find more patches of sun. The life without feeling was a lot less painful, but it was really no life at all. I am beginning to feel empathy and pain – and sometimes joy. But these are closer to being human than to feel nothing at all.

Wayne had feared that exploring his war trauma would uncover feelings that would overwhelm him. He had chosen numbness as a way to survive during the war and afterward. He found, as many others have, that much of what is feared is not as dreadful as it seems when it is finally faced and brought into the light.

Sometimes therapy can be very important in sorting through the confusion of past actions and understanding them in a new and healthier way. This can often change a past demon into something much tamer. Art and Drew are two more examples of men who finally faced dreaded memories from the past and benefited from exploring them in therapy. They needed a therapist at their sides, as they sorted through the confused memories and feelings of their wars, to come to a better understanding of what was the "truth" they had to face.

It was 30 years after Vietnam when I first saw Art. He had spent 18 months in Vietnam, flying over 60 combat missions as a helicopter crew chief and door gunner. Some of those missions were extremely dangerous, including their efforts to re-supply the Marines and extract their wounded when a Marine unit was surrounded in a major North Vietnamese offensive. He was shot down three times. He did his duty and was an honorable soldier.

Ten years after Vietnam, Art began having a recurring and very troubling nightmare. In the nightmare he and his best friend are at their base in a tent. They are hit by a large caliber rocket, wounding Art and throwing him about 30 feet from the tent. He hears his best friend calling for help but ignores him and crawls to safety in a nearby bunker. During the 20 years since the nightmare first occurred, he began to fear that it was really a suppressed memory, and that he had refused to come to his friend's aid but had sought his own safety first. He feared that he had committed a combatant's worst sin – abandoning a comrade at his time of greatest need to seek his own safety. By the time I saw him, he was feeling "eaten alive by this nightmare."

Several aspects of this story troubled me when I first heard it. First, the "memory" didn't begin until ten years after Vietnam. Second, Art and his friend were still in regular contact – contact maintained by his friend. He abandoned a man in his greatest need, and that man still counts him as one of his best friends? Third, how could Art remember anything after being blown 30 feet and knocked unconscious by a rocket blast? The concussion would make accurate memories of the event impossible. Finally, how could he hear his friend calling for help? After getting blasted by a rocket like that, a person can't hear anything for a while.

To my question about the ten years of no memory of this event, Art responded with the usual pop psychiatry: "Well, it was a painful memory of when I was a coward and I must have suppressed it until it surfaced in my dreams."

To my question about why his friend was still his friend when he had abandoned him, Art responded, "I don't think he remembers it that way. He says someone ran by him to the bunker and refused to help him when he was calling for help, but he thinks it was this other guy in the unit. I don't think that's right. I don't think he was there that day, so it must've been me."

When I asked in detail about what he remembered about the incident before the dream began occurring, Art responded, "We were talking in the tent. The next thing I remember is waking up in the bunker being patched up by the medic. I realized we were under rocket attack and asked where Rick was. No one seemed to know, and I yelled that he must be back at the tent. I screamed for someone to go get him and they did."

When I asked him how he got to the bunker, Art admits he doesn't know, but supposes he crawled there.

When I ask about the transient deafness from a rocket blast, Art remembers seeing that happen in the war and cannot explain how he heard Rick call at that point.

This is what I think happened. Both men are in their tent. It is rocketed. Both are wounded and knocked unconscious by the blast. Art either crawls like a dazed animal to the bunker or is carried there by other soldiers. He and Rick come to at about the same time. He is in the bunker when he comes to and Rick is lying wounded somewhere near the tent. When Art realizes Rick is not there and asks about him, men from the bunker go look for Rick and bring him back for treatment. Neither one of them has accurate memories of the event because of the severe concussions they experienced at the time they were wounded.

The nightmare that Art is having is a typical old battle dream that is a familiar mix of truth and imagined horror. The truth is the rocket attack. The fantasy is the brain's attempt to replace the vacuum of the lost time from the concussion with a new memory – a "memory" created from his worst fears. But this memory is no more real than dreaming about weapon barrels melting when they are needed most, or an enemy getting up and coming after you despite filling him full of lead or blowing his head off – both of which are typical of combat nightmares.

I present my interpretation to Art. He finds it hard to accept immediately. He is still struggling with the question, "Is it possible that the nightmare is just that, a nightmare, and not a true memory?" I also suggest that the same is probably true of his friend. He is blaming the innocent. His dreams have probably confused his memories also.

Art was motivated by our discussion to contact Rick again and for the first time discuss this event with him in detail. He found out that his nightmare memories were not accurate. Rick remembers coming to and seeing Art bleeding profusely from a head wound. Rick thought Art was dead and then Art spoke to him. Rick states that just knowing Art was alive gave Rick the will to live. Art's memory of seeing Rick wounded is accurate according to Rick, because Rick spoke with Art. Art then passed out and Art and Rick were both taken to the bunker for medical care. Rick says that when he was brought to the bunker, Art was being held by their door gunner and the medic was treating him. No one was at fault. All did their duties. Art now states:

> That discussion about my nightmare gave me the courage to open up with Rick and get his fuller version of what happened. We have met three times since then and talked it out in great detail. I am so relieved. Our friendship is important to me. That nightmare was eating me up and making me miserable. It is now gone. I have been able to move on to other issues in therapy.

Another subtle example of an emotionally and spiritually damaging misinterpretation of a wartime event involves the WWII airborne vet, Drew (see Chapter 4). He parachuted with his unit behind enemy lines to capture a bridge in "Operation Market Garden" in September 1944. He broke his foot and sprained his ankle, but splinted it and led a group of men to a canal bridge they needed to capture. After dark he climbed an embankment and killed one of the guards silently with a knife. He motioned the other men up, and they went on to surprise the Germans and capture the bridge. His broken foot became impossible to use as it continued to swell. When the British linked up, he was evacuated to England where his foot was operated on. He never returned to combat.

In England Drew replayed what happened over and over. What he couldn't forgive himself for was the feeling of elation that came over him as he slit the teenage German guard's throat. How could any decent human feel elation at a time like that? Later in life, every time he saw his teenage sons he was reminded painfully of that event and his response. When he started to have the same problem with his teenage grandson, he finally came in, but had little faith we could help him. He had talked with a couple of different priests over the years, but it never helped. He still could not forgive himself for his response.

Now this is the rest of the story. Drew was an outstanding welterweight boxer. He represented his division all over England and almost always won. He loved the competition and the challenge. He also was expert in hand-to-hand fighting and taught classes regularly to the men in his division. He could make a fool of a man twice his size. On close questioning, he admitted that the elation he experienced when he killed the young German guard on the embankment was just what he felt when he won a boxing match. My interpretation is that the conditions so closely resembled his experiences in the ring that he was inevitably going to experience elation when he killed the guard, just as if he had won a boxing match in front of his division. The conditioning was so strong that it was his most likely immediate response. Then, as a decent human being, he thought back on this killing and his response and it troubled him. In reality, he felt elation over "winning," not killing. His competitive boxing had conditioned him to have this response.

When presented with this hypothesis, Drew agreed that this reinterpretation was plausible, and it did help him; but it did not immediately reverse the impact of 50 years of self-condemnation and shame. We continue to work on this and other issues, but as he notes now, "I am doing a lot better with this than I was ten years ago when I started therapy. But I still killed a boy masquerading as a soldier with my bare hands." Yet Drew did not put that boy in a uniform and assign him to guard a bridge at night in a battle zone.

We often feel guilty about what we have done without apportioning appropriate responsibility to others for their actions. This irrational sense of responsibility can be an important target of therapy in this circumstance. "I should have been able to," even though it would have been "impossible to" is many times a successful focus of therapy. Rationally processing what was realistically possible and comparing that to what one wished could have happened can prove helpful.

Herb, Luther, Art and Drew were all troubled by shameful memories that did not prove to be as shameful when they finally explored them in detail with therapists and other vets. This is not always the case, but it often is. The interpretation an 18-year-old might give to an event can be very different from that of a mature 50-year-old. Therapy, individual or group, gives the 50-year-old a chance to explore with others the meaning of events that happened during teenage war years. The wisdom of experience and age often softens the harsh self-condemnation of the teenage warrior, when as a mature adult he has the courage to finally face his worst memories and explore them in the light of the present day.

How is facing the truth different from telling the story? In some cases it is not. In Herb's case it was the same. He was the airman from Chapter 6 who blamed himself for failing to rescue his ball-turret gunner. He only had one story to tell that was important to him. When he finally got the courage to talk, after listening in group therapy for two years, he faced his most feared demons as he told the story for the first time. For most vets, though, telling the story is different from facing the truth. They may talk for years before they get the courage to expose their most dreaded fears and begin working on them. Most who have struggled with alcoholism have to begin to face the shame from the alcoholism before they can successfully address their most dreaded events from the war.

How is this different from a religious doctrine like confession? Sometimes there isn't any difference. Often as a therapist I feel like a privileged outsider watching as veterans deal deeply with God and faith. Sometimes they do it privately while we work on other issues, but they trust me enough to share what is going on. Other times they have already done the spiritual work and they are kind enough to fill me in on the details. Confession implies talking with the offended person and seeking forgiveness. Most often those potentially offended are dead or unreachable. Yet while trying to face and conquer their own personal war demons, many men do try to apologize and seek forgiveness from those they feel they have offended. Boyd was doing that when he contacted Guy; and he is still trying to help a Vietnamese family recover the remains of a loved one and give those remains a proper burial.

Sometimes I share what I have seen work for other vets with a troubled vet to get him to consider exploring potentially healing spiritual issues. I might say something like, "The majority of men I have seen successfully work this through have all involved God or what they see as spiritual powers in some way. How might that apply to you?" The beginning of this last phase of spiritual or moral healing always seems to start with having the courage to face the truth no matter how painful and shameful it may seem to be. Once the truth is faced, we can start looking for further understanding and resolution.

At this point have we left the realm of psychiatry? I am not sure what the realm of psychiatry is any more. I have been changed by this work. I see no option many times but to go deeper with my veterans into spiritual and religious realms as they seek the answers they need. I go there now because the majority of those who have recovered the most from their war trauma have taken me into spiritual realms on their own quests for redemption. And I have seen how much more powerful this can be than what we ordinarily do in therapy. When I go there with them, I am not acting as someone who has the answers, but as a supportive human who has watched many men with secret but profound feelings of guilt and shame go on their own spiritual quests and find significant redemption.

Notes

1   Clewell, Richard D., D. Min. "Moral Dimensions in Treating Combat Veterans with Posttraumatic Stress Disorder", *Bulletin of the Menninger Clinic*, January; 51(1):114–130 pp. 117–18.
2   The Centers for Disease Control Vietnam Experience Study. "Postservice Mortality Among Vietnam Veterans" *JAMA* 1987; 257:790–5.
3   Kang, Han K., Dr. P.H., and Tim A. Bullman, M.S., "Mortality Among U.S. Veterans of the Persian Gulf War", *The New England Journal of Medicine*, 1996; 335:1498–504.
4   For a great description of the fighting involving Luther's unit see: Phibbs op. cit. pp. 115–61.

Chapter 15

Mercy, Reparative Acts and Forgiveness

"Blessed are the merciful: for they shall obtain mercy."

Matthew 5:7

Chapter 1 of this book started with several examples of the killing typical of war. I quoted Ed, who saw and participated in just about every type of gruesome war-related killing. It was he who painfully asked in my first WWII combat vets group about two years after it began, "Aren't we all murderers?"

The passage below, written by the WWII combat surgeon Brendan Phibbs, illustrates the response of many soldiers to their first encounter with the "ordinary" killing of war:

I'd been looking out across the field when the first shell exploded next to one of our half-tracks and I'd run out across the field to the shouts of "Medic!" A wounded man was lying across an aid man's knees. His face was streaming red and I foolishly concentrated on it, mopping blood with an aid packet, looking for the lacerations, ignoring the frantic stammering of the aid man. Finally he connected words. "He ain't got no back on his head, Major. It's all tore off at the back." As we turned the boy over his brains slid out on my lap and he died with a couple of agonal gurgles. The occiput was torn off as neatly as if a neurosurgeon had been sawing and chiseling.

The sound of the next shell ripping the air in our direction sent us flat: I sprinted in bursts back to the command post, diving under tanks between explosions, furious, raging with impatience to get to a radio to call appropriate authorities to deal with the criminals who had just torn a boy's skull off.

Old murder was one thing; the cooling dead were something a mind could imbibe, given a shudder, but seeing somebody killed for the first time, actually seeing the body's parts sundered, sent reason squalling into outrage. Since when were people allowed to get away with murder? Before I could shout it at the colonel the question crumpled under the appalling swift answer from subterranean knowledge. Since forever. Since the first primates pulled themselves into clans and began social killing. The truth reared on its hindquarters, waving the bloody claws that only soldiers see, roaring what's only learned on the killing grounds, that murder is what is expected, enforced, required, legal, proper, rewarded. Someone, somewhere, was being patted on the back by appropriate authority for tearing the bones off a boy's brain. To refuse to commit murder, to disclaim any part as an accomplice, is to suffer the punishment of one's proper, God-invoking, white-papered, courtroom-bounded governance.[1]

For many ordinary soldiers, participation in the killing of war creates a burden of guilt that is difficult to face and resolve. This occurs when those they kill are formal enemy combatants. It is even more painful when those killed are civilians, or other friendly combatants, or their comrades, as described in Chapter 4. After facing the reality and pain of having killed or "broken the soldier's trust" in some fashion, how can men then successfully address and resolve their feelings of guilt and shame?

A few years ago I was interviewing a Vietnam vet who was just starting treatment. He had served with the 1st Air Cavalry Division. When questioned about why he was seeking treatment now, he reluctantly and sadly said, "I was a good soldier until my last day there and then I was a coward. Since then I have had a hard time living with myself. I was hoping you might somehow help me."

He had served in Vietnam a little over one year and was twelve days past his official date to leave Vietnam. Men often "sweated out" a few days or weeks of extra combat if their unit was heavily engaged and the paperwork generating their official orders to return to America was delayed. For several months he had been serving as a radio operator and providing covering rifle fire and smoke screens for medics when they went in on medevacs. He acted as their body guard while the medics were picking up and evacuating wounded.

His medevac team started his last day in Vietnam visiting a unit that had captured 33 North Vietnamese soldiers. Just before they arrived, a captured female North Vietnamese medic who had her hands tied behind her back had been "jumping around and wouldn't stay still." For this she had been shot. He went and looked at her. She was lying in her own blood with her hands still tied behind her back. He explained his response to this:

> She looked like a human being, a real person. What had she done to deserve death? We had two more missions that day. Both were hot dust-offs [meaning they were done under enemy fire]. I couldn't shoot my weapon anymore. I couldn't do my job. I was sick and numb. I was a coward. I couldn't kill the enemy. Before, I was always the last man out. I made sure everyone had boarded before me. But on these two missions I tried to board early. On the last

dust-off, I actually tried to walk into enemy fire. One of the medics risked his life to knock me down and drag me to safety. I was supposed to be protecting him, but instead he was nearly killed saving me.

I was still ruminating about this vet and where to go with his treatment as we began a group therapy session with combat vets from WWII, Korea and Vietnam later that same day. I related his story and asked them what they thought it meant and how they would deal with it.

It sparked a powerful but painful discussion about civilian and friendly fire deaths. One vet spoke of shooting at running noises at night on their perimeter while fighting the Japanese on Okinawa. The next morning they found a nine-year-old girl holding her father's head and softly moaning. They had killed her father that night as he was trying to slip between the Japanese and American lines to safety with his daughter. Speaking of his response to this Okinawan's death and the little girl's overwhelming grief, he quietly said, "It was like a dagger to my heart."

Another vet related killing North Vietnamese soldiers while they slept and the soul searching he has gone through ever since. After most had shared their thoughts, one ex-Special Forces officer, Larry, stated the following:

> It was because she was a woman and a medic. He had been trying to protect medics. Now for no rational reason he is looking at a female medic who was shot by our guys while she was tied up. He couldn't stomach it. It was not acceptable that our guys had done this. It was terribly wrong and he knew it. He wasn't a coward. He was just made sick of war and mad at our own men for having killed this helpless female medic. They had done what he tried to keep the North Vietnamese and Vietcong from doing every day – kill defenseless medics.

He then went on and related this story:

> The High Command had planned the first B-52 carpet-bombing raid in Vietnam. I was leading a platoon of former Vietcong who had been recruited by the CIA to fight for us. We had been training together one month when we were assigned to do the BDA [bomb damage assessment] after the bombing. The bombing was designed to destroy two battalions of VC. We were to be put in immediately after the raid, make the assessment, and then be extracted. Because our High Command let the South Vietnamese government and military know about the bombing raids, the VC always knew what was coming and cleared out, or took cover, to avoid the bombs, but we didn't know that at the time. We only realized that later.

When we were put in, we could see that the raid was unsuccessful. All the VC were gone. There were a lot of women and children there, and even they were unhurt. They were all asking to leave with us as we started to pull out. We explained the situation to High Command by radio and were ordered to take them with us. My reformed VC lieutenant and interpreter said we were in trouble. He said the women were just trying to delay us and that this was all a trap. We needed to hustle to the extraction point or we would be ambushed by the VC before we could get out. I knew he was right but had received a direct order to leave with all the women and children. I compromised and took only six women. We scattered the rest by shooting over their heads when they tried to crowd around us.

It all turned out as my lieutenant predicted. When we got to the extraction point, the VC had a mortar and a machine gun zeroed in on the area. We had to call off the extraction birds and bring in gun ships to take out the mortar. We then brought in the choppers again. We were under sporadic fire as we loaded up. The women continued to delay us. As I was getting on the last chopper, one of the women jumped off and started running for the jungle. My lieutenant requested permission to shoot her, saying she was obviously VC and had been in on the ambush. I knew he was probably right, but I couldn't stomach shooting an unarmed woman in the back, and I refused. I had never intentionally shot an unarmed woman, and neither my men nor I ever did.

We were ordered to go in for the next B-52 BDA. This time a Chinese Nung [Chinese born in South Vietnam who fought for the Americans] commando unit was to accompany us to finish off any stunned survivors. As soon as we got there, it smelled like a trap. As we were preparing to leave, we were ambushed. Two of my men went down and I saw a grenade coming towards me. It was as if everything slowed down. As I dove, the grenade exploded. I came down with my automatic weapon trapped under me. I looked up helplessly into the eyes of a VC with an AK-47 pointed at me no more than ten feet away. He looked at me for a moment and then turned and ran off, firing at the Chinese.

We got out. For a while, I tried to tell myself that he didn't shoot me because he thought I was dead. But I had looked right up at him and he had looked right at me. As time has gone on, I have had a stronger and stronger feeling that he didn't shoot me because I hadn't shot that woman in the back the previous mission. It may seem irrational, but that is what I believe.

There was a long pause. Finally I said, "He couldn't have known that?"

He responded, "Oh, of course not."

"Do you mean you received mercy for mercy?"

"Yes, I received mercy for mercy, just like in the Bible. I refused to kill that woman, and when I was helpless, I was spared. That is just how I see it now."

In our hearts we resonate to a cosmic balance. The vets often use the common phrases, "We reap what we sow," or "What goes around comes around." If we are merciful, we have more confidence that we could receive mercy. If we act with love, we might receive the same again. If we forgive, we can start to believe we might be forgiven.

The feelings of most of my vets are loosely or more directly connected with the religious teachings and concepts taught in the Bible. These include ideas such as that referenced by Larry in the preceding paragraph, implying that mercy is received for mercy shown. The hope that "I can be forgiven" comes more readily to the mind and hearts of those who forgive: "For if ye forgive men their trespasses, your heavenly Father will also forgive you: but if ye forgive not men their trespasses, neither will your Father forgive your trespasses."[2]

Larry was right about this vet. At some level that last day, he began to feel that neither he nor his medics deserved to be protected, because Americans from his division had murdered a defenseless female medic. He had felt he was fighting honorably to defend medics from an enemy that had no respect for our Red Crosses. Now his own side seemed to have no respect for a helpless female captive, and where did that leave him? He was left with no hope of mercy. In fact, he felt he deserved death. Maybe they all did. For one day, this atrocity overwhelmed his faithful devotion to his medics. Then, because he failed to do his job in those last two medevacs and even forced one medic to risk death to save him instead of the other way around, he was left with the belief that he had broken their trust in him. Thankfully, none of his medics were killed to add to his burden. In the end he responded well to treatment, as his reactions were explored and understood.

Mercy is the opposite of vengeance. A Vietcong woman tries to lead you to your death in an ambush. When you have the chance, you could exact justice. Instead, you are merciful and spare her. Mercy is not imposing vengeful or retributive justice when you have the opportunity. Mercy is inconsistent with the hate frequently generated by war. Hate and bitterness have to be let go for mercy to have a place.

After shooting down 28 Japanese planes in the Pacific, "Pappy" Boyington was shot down and spent 20 months in Japanese prison camps. He was beaten, humiliated and starved. He should have come out of that experience like many others did, with a burning hatred of the Japanese.

Because Boyington was a well-known Medal of Honor recipient and the Marine Corps' leading ace, the US government sent him on tours after the war to encourage the purchase of war bonds to help finance America's war debts. In his autobiography he notes that he didn't really like speaking to audiences, but did so anyway. "... I felt I had something to say to Americans that was useful. The audience would be disappointed at first, or at least puzzled at first, why I – all banged up by beatings, wounds, and so on – didn't hate the Japanese." He goes on to explain why his audience shouldn't hate them either, essentially saying that if we treat them with respect and mercy now, they can become valuable friends later. He not only delivered this message of mercy, but he firmly believed it. This belief made it possible for him to be receptive to the merciful help he would later need from his second wife, friends, and in his words, "Infinite Wisdom," to recover from his alcoholism and war trauma.[3]

As I have watched vets over the last two decades, I have seen that those who hold onto the hate and who cannot begin to feel mercy for their former enemy, continue to reject the real help they need to recover. The hate keeps the war alive forever.

Talking about his own survival at Auschwitz and his recovery from the Holocaust, Viktor Frankl makes a similar point about his fellow survivors after their liberation:

During this psychological phase one observed that people with natures of a more primitive kind could not escape the influences of the brutality which had surrounded them in camp life. Now, being free, they thought they could use their freedom licentiously and ruthlessly. The only thing that had changed for them was that they were now the oppressors instead of the oppressed. They became instigators, not objects, of willful force and injustice. They justified their behavior by their own terrible experiences. This was often revealed in apparently insignificant events. A friend was walking across a field with me toward the camp when suddenly we came to a field of green crops. Automatically, I avoided it, but he drew his arm through mine and dragged me through it. I stammered something about not treading down the young crops. He became annoyed, gave me an angry look and shouted, "You don't say! And hasn't enough been taken from us? My wife and child have been gassed – not to mention everything else – and you would forbid me to tread on a few stalks of oats!"

Only slowly could these men be guided back to the commonplace truth that no one has the right to do wrong, not even if wrong has been done to them. We had to strive to lead them back to this truth, or the consequences would have been much worse than the loss of a few thousand stalks of oats. I can still see the prisoner who rolled up his shirt sleeves, thrust his right hand under my nose and shouted, "May this hand be cut off if I don't stain it with blood on the day when I get home!" I want to emphasize that the man who said these words was not a bad fellow. He had been the best of comrades in camp and afterwards.[4]

Many combat vets, like Holocaust survivors, feel that wrong has been done to them. They have seen their most beloved friends killed by a seemingly merciless enemy. Many combat vets were POWs under concentration camp-like conditions. But unlike "Pappy" Boyington or Viktor Frankl, they may still breathe out hate for their captors.

At the same time these vets are not just objects of violence and death but also perpetrators of the same. They, too, have killed. They long for mercy, reconciliation and forgiveness. If they let their desire for revenge lead them to further wrongs in combat or later in their lives, they have an even greater need for mercy and reconciliation. If they keep their hate close to their hearts, they never seem to have room for mercy or conciliatory acts. In this state they remain mired in the hate of war.

One farmer I know well, who was a 1st Marine Division vet and a survivor of the vicious fighting on Okinawa, came home with an unbending hatred of the Japanese. He went back to farming but he would buy nothing Japanese. He would talk to no one who looked Japanese. He would watch nothing that depicted the Japanese favorably in any way. He started a family and even attended church. There was a façade of recovery. But he was crippled by his hate. His oldest boy came of age to serve a mission for their church. He received his mission call for two years of service in – Japan!

His father was livid. He threatened not to let him go and not to talk to him if he went. His son went anyway and had a great experience. He wrote home regularly. His dad could not open the letters because they came from Japan. He was in hellish inner turmoil. Eventually a letter came from some Japanese expressing their love for his son and their gratitude to the family for sending their son to help them. At his wife's insistence he finally read this letter, trembling as he did so. Then he started to cry. The tears could not be stopped. When he was done, the hate had washed away and his real recovery from the war began. Through the medium of this letter, he was put in the dilemma of hating people who obviously loved and respected his son. The love of these Japanese for someone he loved so deeply softened his heart. He told me he believed that with his heart softened, God's influence had entered into his soul and filled him with mercy and forgiveness, replacing the hate with peace.

Just as hate can lead to acts of revenge and further misery, mercy usually leads to acts that can start the process of forgiveness, reconciliation and peace. For any individual, these acts can begin even during the war. Many men kill and even kill in large numbers but never let hate become part of who they are. George, mentioned in Chapter 4, was like this. He commanded a US-Filipino guerilla force on Luzon in WWII. He dealt with the Japanese harshly when he had to in order to survive and preserve his men, but he did not kill with hate. Because he didn't let hate control his actions, he was always prepared to be merciful, provided he could do that and still fight the war successfully.

When I read the autobiographical account of Richard O'Kane, I see the same – a man who kills as a duty but never with hate. He was responsible for the deaths of thousands of Japanese as he led his submarine, the *Tang*, on some of the most successful patrols of WWII. Yet in his book he expresses sadness for the men he killed as his submarine efficiently accomplished the duty for which it and the men manning it were commissioned – to destroy Japanese shipping.

O'Kane took great joy and pride in one mission where they didn't sink any Japanese ships. Instead, they repeatedly surfaced and risked their lives to rescue 22 USN airmen off Truk when their sub was assigned lifeguard duty during a naval air assault on this major Japanese base. This is an example of a reparative act – saving life instead of taking it.

On that mission, as described in O'Kane's book, we also meet Lieutenant J.A. Burns, who contributed mightily to these 22 rescues. He landed his Kingfisher floatplane inside Truk Lagoon and braved Japanese fire to drag eight airmen to safety by taxiing them out of the lagoon to be picked up by the *Tang*. He did this until his own plane was no longer serviceable. It is easy to see how much O'Kane admired this young ensign's heroism as they worked together to save lives rather than to take them.[5]

Burns flew off the battleship *North Carolina*. I have often wondered if he was still on the *North Carolina* a year later when my patient witnessed one Kingfisher pilot rescuing another under similar circumstances. If he was there, was he the rescued or the rescuer? (See the beginning of Chapter 13.)

Rescuing others is a powerful reparative act. It can have even more healing power than simply watching or being the recipient of others' heroics as related in the antidote experiences of Chapter 13. Personally taking reparative action gives the soldier more hope that he can receive mercy and maybe even forgiveness. A 1st Marine Division vet reminded me of this when I treated him for several months shortly before his death. He was dying of cancer and had no family left. After hearing about my WWII veterans group, he asked to attend until he died. Although he had been through the horrific experience of Guadalcanal, he was not particularly troubled by his war experiences any longer. In group he was consistently supportive of the other men. Once, we got him to tell us what he remembered most about Guadalcanal. He was shy about talking, but he finally admitted he was most proud of the two wounded airmen he rescued.

Iron Bottom Sound is the treacherous, shark-infested strait between Guadalcanal and Tulagi. The Marine airmen who flew out of Henderson Field on Guadalcanal were often the only force that kept the US Marines on Guadalcanal from being overrun by the Japanese. This vet was an excellent swimmer. On two occasions when wounded airmen parachuted into the Sound, he swam out to them and brought them ashore. Because of the thousands of sailors killed in the Sound, the sharks were accustomed to eating humans. He knew that, yet he swam out without hesitation, sometimes as far as one mile into the Sound, and brought back men as they bled into the water. When asked, "Why?" his only response was, "I was a good swimmer and they needed me."

George Patton describes a medic with a similar attitude:

On the sixth, I decorated Private Harold A. Garman, of the 5th Infantry Division, with the Medal of Honor. Garman was an attached medico in one of the battalions that forced the crossing over the Sauer River. During the action, a boat with three walking and one prone wounded, paddled by two engineers, started back and was caught by German machine-gun fire in the middle of the river. The engineers, and one of the walking wounded, jumped overboard and swam for shore. The other two wounded jumped overboard, but were too weak to swim and clung to the boat while the litter case lay prone. The boat, still under a hail of bullets, drifted toward the German shore. Private Garman swam out and pushed the boat to our side. I asked him why he did it, and he looked surprised and said, "Well, someone had to."[6]

Actions such as these make a combatant feel that there is the possibility of mercy and even forgiveness for the killings he may have done.

Often more important are the attitudes and convictions that guide men to take reparative action after the war. We previously discussed the case of Boyd (see Chapter 9). Guided by the cleansing principles of Native American "sweats" and AA, he tried to make direct amends to the people he felt he had harmed most both in the war and while an active alcoholic. He was seeking to apologize to and ask forgiveness from Guy (Steps Eight and Nine of AA) when he had his joyous and healing reunion with him. By that point, because of his efforts to forgive and make amends, he was fully receptive to the healing spiritual force of forgiveness and reconciliation he discovered in his reunion with Guy.

A few years ago I watched the movie *The Patriot*. I hoped to see an honest portrayal of the life and war experiences of the man many consider the father of successful guerilla warfare, Revolutionary War hero Francis Marion. Instead I saw another Hollywood combat fantasy. It did motivate me, though, to try to discover the real Francis Marion. His most definitive biographer was Hugh Rankin. In that biography I found portrayed a man who suffered through all the usual war traumas and moral dilemmas my vets confront over two hundred years later. I was impressed with his post-war recovery and life, and saw in it all the signs of a man who understood and acted on the principles of truth, mercy and forgiveness.

While Marion was serving in the South Carolina Senate after the war, a bill was proposed exempting officers like him from litigation from those who alleged they had been wronged during the war. Marion vehemently opposed this legislation even though it would have been a great protection to him. Despite his opposition it passed, but he refused to allow his name to be listed with those exempted from litigation. He stated:

> If I have given any occasion for complaint, I am ready to answer in property and person. If I have wronged any man I am willing to make him restitution. If, in a single instance, in the course of my command, I have done that which I cannot fully justify, Justice requires that I should suffer.[7]

He was willing to face any unpleasant truth about himself in the name of justice.

To the surprise of many, Marion was completely supportive of accepting the Loyalists back into the full life of the community. His mercy in this regard was constantly evident despite the many bitter battles he had with them during the war. He sponsored bills favorable to the Loyalists and requested the legislators "not to sully their minds with thoughts of retaliation." Soon after the end of the war, when a Loyalist petitioned the Assembly for a pardon, Marion was very supportive of this "prayer for forgiveness." He declared, "God has given us victory. Let us show our gratitude to Heaven, which we shall not do by cruelty to man."[8]

Marion remained supportive of all his old war comrades. They could count on him for loyalty and friendship, but only if they followed the law and helped establish the peace.[9] He returned to the hard work of farming and finally married a like-tempered woman. He was of service to his community and others throughout his life. Rankin notes, "He was a good citizen, performing those tasks in the community for which he felt he was qualified."[10] Rankin sums up by saying of Marion, "His emotional conflicts were great, yet he was able to temper the cruelty of war with the compassion of peace."[11]

The pattern of Marion's post-war life – his willingness to face the truth about himself and his actions during the war, his mercy overcoming any bitterness he may have had, his acts of reparative service, and his willingness to forgive – is a recipe that can lead to inner peace for combatants. After their wars, the combat vets I see who are coping best lead lives of service. Many work as fire fighters, policemen, teachers, emergency medical technicians, and in other medical services. Some are devoted Alcoholics Anonymous sponsors – helping others find the strength through AA fellowship to change their lives. They are involved in their religions as lay ministers and in making their communities better places through organized charities and their own acts of goodness. It isn't that these acts necessarily "balance the scales of justice," but I do see these acts making these men more receptive to human and divine powers of healing. Acts of love leave little room for hate. Mercy enters in. Where mercy enters in, understanding and forgiveness soon follow. If veterans can forgive their enemy, then they can start believing that they may be forgiven also. At this point men like Ed (see Chapter 1) can start to become receptive to the idea that they can recover spiritually, even from the "murders" of war.

Notes

1   Phibbs op. cit. pp. 80–1.
2   Bible, Matthew 6:14–15, KJV.
3   Boyington, Gregory "Pappy", *Baa Baa Black Sheep*, pp. 351–2.
4   Frankl, Victor, *Man's Search for Meaning*, pp. 112–13.
5   O'Kane, Richard H., *Clear the Bridge*, p. 165.
6   Patton op. cit. p. 270.
7   Rankin, Hugh, *Francis Marion: The Swamp Fox*, p. 291.
8   Ibid p. 292.
9   Ibid pp. 294–5.
10 Ibid p. 295.
11 Ibid p. 299.

Chapter 16

Spiritual Connection and Recovery

"You have to give up even justified bitterness and hate to fully heal the emotional and spiritual wounds of war."

Larry, a retired professional soldier

I initially treated Al for depression shortly after I started working at the Boise VAMC. He had a significant family history of the disease. He responded well to medication and his depression remained in remission as long as he took his anti-depressant. I knew he had served in WWII, but he had no obvious symptoms of PTSD, so I did not explore it deeply with him in our initial work together. As I learned more about the war and PTSD from my other vets, I started to question Al about where he served and what he did. I was surprised to discover he had served with the infantry in New Guinea. I knew there had been many grim and merciless battles there with the Japanese.[1] I discovered that he had been in some of the worst.

At one point I wondered aloud why he seemed so little troubled by his war experiences. He teased that he would tell me the full truth if I promised not to lock him up. I promised and he shared the following:

I was in the signal corps. My job was to keep the phone lines between the company and battalion headquarters open and functioning. This was no easy task in the intense fighting. Wires could be cut by infiltrators or blasted in artillery barrages. Often phones needed to be replaced. This put me on the move and exposed me to enemy fire.

I was at a company CP [command post] in the middle of a nasty fight when the phone went dead to battalion. I tested the phone, but it did not seem to be the problem. Assuming the wire had been cut, I started to follow it back to battalion HQ [headquarters] as cautiously as I could. I was maybe halfway there when I found the break and the reason for the break at the same time. The line had been cut by artillery fire as it crossed an open area. Just as I started to patch it, I suspect the Japanese spotted me, because I was caught in a fresh artillery barrage. I have never been so terrified in my life. It was deafening. I was completely exposed and was bouncing up and down, face down, in the dirt with each explosion. I must have been screaming to God, for I heard in the midst of the barrage a voice say as quietly and distinctly as you talking to me now, "You will survive the war." The barrage continued, but I felt completely at peace and never doubted God had spoken to me. I vowed to live a good life from then on and find out as much as I could about God. I have kept my word. War held no terror for me after that. I did my duty to the end.

I had no reason to question Al's story. He was sincere in believing that he had been touched and preserved by God and that God had spoken to him. This experience and his religious involvement after the war had certainly helped him cope with his war trauma. Except for his depression, he had done very well.

A few years later I was reading E.B. Sledge's autobiographical account of his time with the 1st Marine Division in the South Pacific in WWII. I was surprised to find the following description of an event that occurred three days into his first combat action on Peleliu. During a brief break in the fighting, he was having a quiet conversation about courage and fear with "Hillbilly," who was one of the most respected officers in his company, Sledge's platoon leader, and the recipient of a battlefield commission on Guadalcanal. As the conversation concludes Sledge describes the following event:

> As the conversation trailed off, we sipped our joe in silence.
>
> Suddenly, I heard a loud voice say clearly and distinctly, "You will survive the war!"
>
> I looked first at Hillbilly and then at the sergeant. Each returned my glance with a quizzical expression on his face in the gathering darkness. Obviously they hadn't said anything.
>
> "Did y'all hear that?" I asked.
>
> "Hear what?" they both inquired.
>
> "Someone said something," I said.
>
> "I didn't hear anything. How about you?" said Hillbilly, turning to the sergeant.
>
> "No, just that machine gun off to the left."
>
> Shortly the word was passed to get settled for the night. Hillbilly and the sergeant crawled back to their hole as Snafu returned to the gun pit. Like most persons, I had always been skeptical about people seeing visions and hearing voices. So I didn't mention my experience to anyone. But I believed God spoke to me that night on that Peleliu battlefield, and I resolved to make my life amount to something after the war.[2]

I was curious how Al would respond to E.B. Sledge's account, so I copied it and handed it to him at our next meeting. His response was typically low key: "Looks like God said the same thing to him he said to me. Except in my case he had to talk a little louder because of the artillery barrage. I hope it helped him as much as it did me."

E.B. Sledge reports that he "... didn't mention my experience to anyone." Al admitted he had never talked about it with anyone before telling me. There is some reluctance on the part of men to discuss these sacred and unusual experiences, but the more I have been open and receptive to hearing about spiritual experiences from vets, the more they have been willing to share them with me. I have found that many combatants report experiences like this, where they describe being guided or reassured by what they consider to be divine forces from outside themselves.[3] These experiences in combat then become a positive force in their recovery and adaptation on returning home. They find prayer and this same type of spiritual comfort uplifting and healing after the war.

Some of my patients and certain authors report that combatants have come to them with just the reverse experience of Al and Sledge. Men feel warned that they will die, but they proceed to do their duty, despite these powerful spiritual premonitions, and are killed as they do so.[4,5,6] I also know of at least one case where a man had a "premonition of impending death" that did not materialize.[7]

Gary, a Vietnam medic (see Chapters 8 and 11), who describes himself as "a Christ believing, yoga practicing, Hindu spiritualist," told me that a Divine voice told him he would be wounded on the day his senior medic and mentor would be sent home. He heard this voice "inside" his head about a month before the events of that day. It all occurred as he had been told. Even though he has been helped by years of treatment, he will tell anyone who asks that the two things that have helped him most since the war have been the companionship and support of other vets and the spiritual comfort and peace he finds in meditation:

Sometimes I am too angry or upset to meditate successfully. Then I need to either talk it through with a good friend or just isolate until I get control of my emotions enough to make good use of the meditation. Then through meditation I can achieve the peace that helps me the most.

Some of the stories I have heard from men in this regard verge on the hilarious, because they are so unusual. Tommy was an infantryman who saw combat in New Guinea, Morotai, Leyte and Luzon in the South Pacific. He was wounded three times, decorated with the Silver and Bronze Stars for bravery, and given a battlefield commission. Toward the end of the war he was in his foxhole during a sharp firefight with the Japanese. He felt God was nudging him to get up and run around his foxhole:

> I responded immediately and started running around the foxhole with the Japs shooting at me. As I was running around, a mortar round landed right in the hole and exploded. Then I jumped back in. If I hadn't responded to that prompting immediately, that mortar round would have killed me. I was kidded by everyone who saw my antics for the rest of the war, but I knew God had warned me and my quick response to that nudging had spared me.

If I had seen Tommy under those circumstances, I also would have been convinced he had finally "cracked" rather than believed he was responding to a life-saving prompting from God!

Although all the men I have quoted above felt aided by these spiritual manifestations, they still struggled with severe symptoms upon returning from their wars. What they did have after the war was a conviction that there were spiritual powers that could help them, through the medium of prayer and meditation.

Larry, who served two and a half years in Southeast Asia and Vietnam as an officer in the US Special Forces, reports: "I prayed every day for protection for my men and myself. I knew my prayers were answered many times, and probably many more times I still don't appreciate. I continue to pray to Christ every day and be guided and supported by Him."

Larry firmly believes that his prayers and spiritual connection with God helped him in four specific ways in Vietnam. He calls these the "fruits" of his prayers and spiritual relationship with God. His use of the word fruits refers to this quote from Matthew 7:16 in the Bible: "Ye shall know them by their fruits. Do men gather grapes of thorns or figs of thistles?" The first fruit was calmness in the chaos of battle: "Praying would calm my mind and allow me to make much better decisions when all hell was breaking loose. It helped me keep my emotions and actions under control when it appeared others might lose control. The calmness I received from God seemed to also reassure my men."

The second and third "fruits" were closely linked. Larry felt that the second fruit was receiving greater wisdom "to make the right choices when planning operations." He saw the third fruit as being able to keep the welfare of his men foremost in his mind when making and executing these battle plans. He acknowledges that their missions were always dangerous:

> But with thorough, wise planning and execution, we always seemed to find a way to accomplish the mission and keep my men alive in doing so. I knew that

if I didn't feel good about a mission, it was a whisper from God. I then needed to review the plan and consider other options until I came up with a plan and options for various contingencies that I was comfortable with.

He acknowledges that some thought he was too cautious, "No one ever said it specifically, but it seemed some American officers wondered why I was so concerned about the lives of my reformed VC and Chinese mercenaries."

The fourth "fruit" was a healthy perspective on the vanity of pursuing "glory, publicity, and body counts." As he explains:

Prayer and my dependence on Christ kept me humble. I knew my success was based on His help. I never felt that drive for fame and recognition that seemed to lead some men into reckless glory hunting. I had a Master to please that did not think glory based on body counts was meaningful. I wanted to accomplish the mission with as little killing as necessary.

Nonetheless killing is often a necessary part of war: "I carry the memory of having brought in air strikes and artillery on the North Vietnamese and Vietcong that killed many hundreds of men. Napalm and massed artillery are horrible but effective weapons of war."

Despite his faith, after the war Larry's use of alcohol to relieve tension, help him sleep, and suppress nightmares got out of hand:

Heavy drinking was an accepted mode of coping and relaxing for most of the officers I associated with, particularly those with significant combat time. I was so angry and drink so seductive that I just didn't see the destructive "fruits" of alcohol in my life. The drinking began to isolate me from my family and threaten my marriage. My wife tried to make me see reason, but I wasn't listening. Finally she said, "I love you, but I can't live with the drinking. You stop or I am leaving and taking the children with me." I knew she meant it. There were a few officers I respected who were teetotalers. They had been leaving literature about A.A. on my desk. I tried to stop on my own but kept failing. I began praying for help just as sincerely as I had in the war. I started attending A.A. and trying to work the program. Because of my wife's toughness and with help from God and the A.A. fellowship, I was finally able to get and stay sober. I am grateful to my wife and those men who persisted until I listened. I am grateful to God for giving me the will power to quit and his merciful help and patience with me throughout my life.

During his last tour in Vietnam, Larry was leading a reconnaissance unit assigned to support a regular army division. He was returning in a Huey after dropping off a small recon team when they received an open radio request for a medevac from a company that had just been ambushed and had taken heavy casualties.

He realized their chopper was the only one available that could get there quickly enough to get the most seriously wounded to the hospital in time to save them. They went in under fire and filled the helicopter with casualties. As they flew off, Larry held one young teenager who had lost both legs. This boy soldier sobbed for his mother until he died in Larry's arms. It affected him deeply:

> I ended my time in Vietnam angry and bitter. I saw so many good young people killed and wounded unnecessarily and foolishly. I blamed the enemy, but even more so I blamed our own military command and politicians for glory hunting and the stupid policies that got so many young men like this killed. What I found, though, was that holding on to that bitterness and hate keeps the wounds open. You have to give up even justified bitterness and hate to fully heal the emotional and spiritual wounds of war. God can help you do this, but you have to help yourself too. You have to keep working on this in therapy. The memories never disappear. The anger can be reactivated by current events. You have to keep praying and getting help to stay on track. I cannot do it on my own. I need continued therapy as well as prayer to keep from slipping back into anger.

Larry, like many other veterans, could only find peace after the war by developing a partnership with God that gave him the strength to lay aside his anger and bitterness and move toward healing, while using appropriate therapy at the same time.

"Pappy" Boyington's story has some similarities to Larry's. Like Larry, he was an older, unorthodox but successful combatant. Like Larry, when he returned from war, alcohol abuse began to wreak havoc in his life and frustrate his chances for a successful post-war adjustment. After divorce from his first wife, the loss of many jobs, failed psychiatric treatments and many public embarrassments due to his drinking, he finally accepted some help:

> Many an early morning when I arrived home by taxicab I discovered that somebody had slipped religious literature into my pockets while I was blacked out. But I wanted no part of religion. I feared that religion would make me so pure if it cured my drinking that I would never want to do anything I considered pleasant.

Somewhere in the back of my mind I had hopes that science would someday develop a pill, or something, to make me a social drinker like other people. Finally I came to the conclusion that I had about as much chance of becoming a social drinker as I would in starting a new political party in the Kremlin. I resigned from the brewery in the spring of 1955 because I was sick and tired of drinking and everything that goes with it.

A few days after this two well-known men whom I knew only by names and pictures dropped over to my home and had a long chat with me. They had had problems with alcohol at one time, but both of them had been sober and happy for years. I listened to their stories and somehow thought they had lived part of my life.[8]

Boyington began attending A.A. with these men and remained sober for several months. He admits that he felt so good that he decided that he could drink again. The result was a "black-out" and waking up nude and ill in a strange bed. He describes the effect of this last relapse on the rest of his life:

This was it! As soon as I could get some coffee down, I was back to my sober drunk friends, willing to do business their way. I asked: "How can I stay sober and happy?"

"You have to progress spiritually, otherwise you will drink again."

"How on earth is a guy like me ever going to progress spiritually, I'd like to know?"

"By meeting with us each week, and helping others to stay sober."

This happened pretty close to three years ago and I haven't had a drink since, simply because I like their way of life a lot better than I ever thought I liked to drink. Otherwise there would be absolutely no reason for living the way I am.

In my lengthy career of violence and fighting this was the first time I ever won by being counted out – by admitting to myself that I was powerless – for a change.

As I live my life from day to day as best I can, past character defects rise to the surface, and I am now able to understand and cope with them. And I find myself gradually joining up with society – something to which I never belonged in my past life.

With the weight of the obsession to drink removed I find that I have time now to appreciate some wonderful things I never thought about before. For an example, birds have always held my interest, but now, when I watch them fly, I think of the Infinite Wisdom telling the birds to fly south before the first snow appears. They know exactly the course to the best feeding, even if they have never been there ...[9]

Larry and Boyington are not unique. Al, Boyd, Guy, JR, Roland, Jed, Norm, Ray, Luther, Doug and many others I have treated would assure anyone who asked that one of the biggest factors in their successful coping with war trauma has been their spiritual partnership with God.

Guy (see Chapter 9) lost both legs and most of his right hand in Vietnam. He faced a nearly overwhelming adjustment as he tried to make a new life for himself after the war:

> My partnership with God kept me alive. When I awoke from the coma induced by my wounds and surgeries, the first person I saw in Da Nang was a nurse from my hometown. I felt God brought her there to give me the courage to live. I promised her I would see her at home in a year at church, and I would be walking. God helped me keep that promise. I prayed constantly. I would ask for the strength to overcome the hurdle in front of me at that time. I would feel peace and strength from God. Each time I got over the hurdle, it gave me greater faith to get over the next. I learned that God answers the prayers of anyone who says, "I can't do this without you. I need your help." All they needed was to have the courage to keep trying and asking and receiving the help God would send in the form of His other children.

Norm describes his partnership with God in these simple but powerful terms:

> For 27 years after my marriage I watched the good effect my wife's religion had on her and my children. After my son returned from a two-year mission, I finally joined their church and stopped drinking. I have learned what prayer can do for you. It has helped me a lot of times. I pray for my wife, my family, myself and many more things. I feel God answering my prayers. Prayer eases my mind and calms me. When you start reading the Bible regularly, it takes your mind away from hate and bitterness and puts your mind where it should be. The scriptures and church have changed my heart. I've even come around to not hating the Japanese.

Another example is the ex-medic, Roland. He feels he has had a long, turbulent, but life-saving partnership with God. He admits that starting with his first firefight, he found himself praying every day. It was a simple prayer of "Save me, God." He would say it each time there was a man down that he had to get to and help:

> I knew the wounded needed me. It seemed there was never a safe way to get to them. I would grab my medical kit and pray as I sprinted or crawled toward them. I hoped God loved them enough to keep me alive. After being wounded a few times myself, I stopped expecting to live, but I didn't stop saying that prayer. I knew my Mom kept praying for me also, and I hoped God would

listen to her, if not me. I had R&R [rest and recovery leave] in the middle of my tour in Hawaii. My girl joined me there. The day I returned to Vietnam I told her I didn't love her, because I loved her so much I didn't want her waiting for a dead man. I guess she didn't believe me because she kept writing and waiting.

A few months later our battalion was heavily engaged with an NVA [North Vietnamese Army] regiment. We were driven back and had to leave some of our dead. Three days later after regrouping and being re-supplied, we counterattacked to recover the ground and the bodies. I could see a body and thought I saw it move. I was sprinting to get to him when a heavy machine gun cut loose. I tripped on the only piece of barbed wire I encountered in Vietnam. It gave me a nasty cut on my shin but saved my life. As I fell heavily on my face the machine gun sawed the banana tree in front of me in half just about waist high. I felt God had tripped me to save me from the fate of the banana tree.

I eventually found one of our abandoned "dead" alive that day. He had been wounded multiple times in the arms and legs and had been unable to retreat with the rest of us. He said, "After you all left, the NVA came around shooting each soldier right in the ass. If the body flinched they gave him a full dose of lead. I closed my eyes and asked God to help me not flinch. Somehow He gave me the strength to take an AK-47 round right in the asshole and never twitch. I have been praying that you would come back looking for us ever since." He was terribly weak and covered with leeches, but I patched him up as best I could and got him out. Maybe his prayers had kept me alive that day. One week later my leg had gotten so infected and swollen from that barbed wire gash that it resembled a tree trunk. I had a high fever and I was evacuated to a field hospital and then a base hospital. I was delirious for a while, but when I came to the man smiling at me in the bed next to mine was the "dead man" I found after the barbed hand of God spared my life.

By the time I had finished in Vietnam I was very angry. Once the guys brought me an NVA to sew up who had his scalp laid open to the bone by a blow from a rifle butt. I sewed him up, but I never used any Novocaine on him. I wanted to make sure I had enough for our guys. It was a mean and ugly thing to do. It shows how mad I was. Our unit wiped out a village. I don't think we had to, but we did it just the same to get at the enemy. Maybe we were all mad just like me. When I came home I was too angry to pray any more. I didn't attend church either. I wasn't angry with God, but the anger was there and it formed a barrier between us. My girl and I married. Her letters had meant so much to me in Vietnam. An old WWII combat surgeon took me under his wing. He convinced me to get training as a nurse. I have kept taking care of people ever since: nursing, EMT, critical care, and now chiropractic medicine. When we started having kids, I knew I had to close the gap between God and I. Some of the anger had receded. I returned to church and I started simple prayers and meditation again. I realized I had been praying all along; I just did it mostly by trying to help others.

As discussed previously, Roland eventually reconnected with another "dead man," the captain he had tied together with bootlaces and evacuated (Chapter 9). He was sure this good officer had died and had been added to the list of men he had tried but failed to save. He describes how finding his captain alive made him feel:

> When I picked up the phone and the Captain said, "My God, Doc, I can't believe I'm talking to the guy who saved my life," I knew God had truly heard my prayers and answered them. I felt God was talking to me through my Captain. I feel reborn and redeemed. The hate and anger are gone. I don't see how life could be sweeter.

Some seem to find God during the war. Others seem to lose God in the war or feel estranged from God by their war experiences. Yet many of the latter in one way or another find that some type of spiritual connection, or reconciliation with God, is a necessary part of their recovery. To make that spiritual connection, most have to begin giving up unjustified and even justified anger and bitterness. They also have to be willing to try to approach God even though they feel significant guilt about the many types of killings they have been involved in.

Doug felt completely estranged from God on returning from Korea (Chapters 1 and 10). He had killed many, and at one point he wrote me that the reason he was afraid to get off the boat in San Francisco on coming home was, "... I had left my poor soul in Korea! THAT'S NOT GOOD!" (emphasis by Doug). He became an alcoholic, and even though he knew it was killing him, he couldn't stop. Thirty years after he returned, in a brief period of sobriety, he heard a voice say:

> "You have not kept the promise you made in Korea."
> What promise? And then I remembered that in the middle of a hellish battle when I was sure I was going to be killed, I had promised God that if he would get me out of this, I would live decently the rest of my life. I knew this reminder came from God, and this experience jolted and scared me so much that I got sober. It has been 20 years since and I have not had a drop.

Doug states that he has, "prayed daily ever since." He has volunteered in prisons and has been active in his church's lay ministry. "I have tried to help others avoid the mistakes I have made and find the same help God has given me." He has quietly attended group therapy now for almost six years, working on his war trauma issues and helping others work on theirs. He is beginning to feel there may be real forgiveness available to him. "Maybe God and all those I killed can forgive me in the end."

Viktor Frankl shares the experience that he considers started his recovery from the physical, emotional and spiritual trauma of Auschwitz:

> One day, a few days after liberation, I walked through the country past flowering meadows, for miles and miles, toward the market town near the camp. Larks rose to the sky and I could hear their joyous song. There was nothing but the wide earth and sky and the lark's jubilation and the freedom of space. I stopped, looked around, and up to the sky – and then I went down on my knees. At that moment there was very little I knew of myself or of the world – I had but one sentence in mind – always the same: "I called to the Lord from my narrow prison and He answered me in the freedom of space."
>
> How long I knelt there and repeated this sentence memory can no longer recall. But I know that on that day, in that hour, my new life started. Step for step I progressed, until I again became a human being.[10]

These experiences may sound unusual and foreign to some, but I find their "fruits" too compelling to discount. For some vets, spiritual connection does not seem to be a major part of their recovery process (for example, Roland's "Captain" in Chapter 9), but for many more it is key. Many times I have heard men avow with deep sincerity, when I have given them the chance, that their personal spiritual experiences and religious faith have been the bedrock on which they have built their recovery from the war. Probably because of the setting and culture around Boise, most of these believers use Christian terminology and find strength in their Christian faiths (Catholic, Mormon, Protestant and others). But others I have worked with have used Yoga, Native American sweats, Jewish traditions, meditation and Alcoholics Anonymous to achieve a sense of spiritual connectedness. The bottom line for these men seems to be their own personal experiences and involvement with what they see as divine and healing forces. All in some way talk of giving up anger, bitterness and hate. All speak of divine spiritual forces touching their hearts and souls. All talk of work and service. These are the actions and powers that lead to the spiritual alchemy of hard, angry, blaming hearts becoming merciful, forgiving and peaceful.

I see it now as an essential part of therapy that I respectfully inquire about veterans' spiritual experiences and beliefs. This exploration allows me to learn about an aspect of their lives that is often key in their recovery and healing. As I am educated by them, this process of discovery often reinforces their healing – accentuating the positive steps they are making in their recovery from war's version of hell.

I see the case of Jed (Chapter 3) as illustrating the major points of this and the previous two chapters. In several months of fighting he lost men he was closer to than he was to most of his family. He was wounded, captured, stripped of his overcoat and boots and abandoned to die by the Red Chinese when his unit was overrun in Korea in February 1951. He was kept alive for a month by a Korean farmer who brought him water and pot scrapings. Jed was then liberated in an American counterattack. When he returned home, he was troubled by the killing he had done. He was bitter and even wished he had killed the American who had surrendered next to him, causing a chain reaction of surrender that resulted in Jed being shot and captured. After his hospitalization and discharge, Jed worked as a farm laborer and drank heavily to suppress his nightmares and numb his feelings. He was a psychological casualty of war with all the symptoms of PTSD and showing no signs of recovery.

Three years after his discharge, Jed met and married his current wife. Their love motivated him to seek education and a better job. Having children caused an even greater change:

> The birth of my first daughter sobered me up. Here was a tiny creature I could totally love. Somehow she softened my heart. I said to myself, "My God, I've got to get my life in order." I stopped drinking. It was hard but love motivated me and I did it. I also forced myself to stop thinking about the war. Every day I would get up and thoughts of the war would just start bubbling up. I made myself think about other things. I concentrated on the needs of the here and now and worked hard. This was a turning point for me. I seemed to recover enough from the war to make a decent life for my family and myself.

Thirty years after the war Jed sought psychological treatment for the first time. He notes, "It had been 30 years of not sleeping. I didn't sleep even after I stopped drinking. I was tired and struggling with depression." Medication and group therapy provided some relief, but the killing he had done bothered him deeply:

> I had helped kill or killed directly a lot of North Korean and Chinese soldiers. I didn't hate them. They came from poor families just like me. The killing you have done disturbs you even more after you have a family. You see then how bad the killing really is. I still hated that American, though, who started the surrendering. I still blamed myself for not shooting him when he first stood and put up his hands. Finally I realized that I would have blamed myself just as much

now if I had shot him. As I prayed about it, I could see that shooting him would have been even worse for me. I am not sure I could have ever lived with myself.

As my children grew up I began praying again. I couldn't understand why God had kept me alive. I knew that after being shot in both lungs, stripped of my coat and boots, and abandoned, that I should have died. I knew only God could have kept me alive. Why was I saved? I started praying and railing at God, "Why did you save me!? What did You keep me alive for!?" I had been praying like this for twenty years. A little over a year ago I was carrying groceries into the house when I heard a voice in my head say, "Love Me." I knew God wanted me to love Him. I knew it meant living a life that was pleasing to God by helping others all I could and doing good with all the blessings I had received. God allowed those words to sound in my head, and my heart rejoiced. I felt I finally knew what God wanted from me. I keep trying to contact the men I served with. I help them when I can. I look for anything I can do to help others that is sensible and reasonable. The hate and bitterness are all gone. I don't blame myself any more.

Jed had no purpose initially after the war. Love for his family and their love for him gave him purpose and the motivation to live and work and get sober. He was still deeply troubled by what he had gone through and done. Group therapy and medication provided some insight and symptomatic relief. His spiritual yearnings, reflected by his diligence in prayer, resulted in a spiritual connection with the Divine. This spiritual connection helped him to abandon bitterness and hate and to feel he could forgive others and himself. This brought him peace and put him on a path of service and altruism that has further reinforced his healing.

The men I treat have participated in every kind of killing: the enemy, civilians and friendly troops. Often grief, pain and guilt have spawned anger and bitterness in their hearts. They carry the burden of the killing, the burden of the deep losses and the burden of the conditioning of war. Many times on top of all this rests the weight of alcohol and drug abuse, and guilt and sadness over the way they treated their families when they were most symptomatic and abusing substances.

These veterans have started to come out from under these burdens by seeking help – often from each other or a loved one, often from professionals like myself, and often from God or some source they see as divine. Usually they need all three. There is a humility that comes from asking for help and receiving it. Some of the anger has to be given up. Some bitterness must be let go. Any recovery starts with facing at least part of the truth about yourself and taking some responsibility for your recovery.

At some point mercy starts to enter in as some of the hate slips away. Sometimes it happens slowly, and sometimes it seems like a miracle as it happens in a rush. Men begin to take reparative action and think about forgiveness. As they act with mercy and forgiveness, they begin to believe they might receive the same. As they persevere in this upward spiral of treatment and recovery, the good builds on the good. Sometimes there are relapses, but more often, once they taste the hope of redemption, men press on, weaving love back into their lives through family, friends, prayer and service.

Insight and understanding moves one toward mercy. Mercy pushes out hate and gives hope of forgiveness. Forgiveness makes room for true reconciliation and peace. At some point combatants can say like Fred (Chapter 10), "I hope for mercy." As the process continues, there is hope that in the end they will be able to say like Roland, "I feel redeemed."

Notes

1 Mayo, Lida, *Bloody Buna*, pp. 193–4, 198–201.
2 Sledge op. cit. pp. 93–4.
3 Recently a WWII Navy vet was referred to me for treatment due to difficulty sleeping. Will was having nightmares of the war reactivated by recent traumatic events – the September 11, 2001 World Trade Center destruction. He had just turned 18 and was serving on the cruiser *New Orleans* when the Japanese attacked Pearl Harbor. He saw much death and destruction that day at Pearl. He was involved in the Battle of the Coral Sea, where he saw the aircraft carrier *Lexington* sunk. His ship rescued hundreds of men from the *Lexington* – most of them seriously burnt – almost all of whom died. They were constantly playing "Taps" and sending those men over the side. The *New Orleans* escorted the carrier *Yorktown* back to Pearl and on to the Battle at Midway, where he saw the *Yorktown* heavily damaged and evacuated. His ship then fought in several major and deadly actions in the Solomon Islands near and around Guadalcanal. In late 1942 or early 1943 the *New Orleans* was returning to Pearl when the following occurred:

> I had begun to worry that I would soon be killed. I couldn't see how I could possibly survive many more battles. I had good eyes and was posted as lookout on the highest point on the ship. I was alone. There was only room for one in that crow's nest. I felt I was as close to God as I could be – up there with the beautiful sky and vast ocean all around. I began praying, pleading with God that I might be spared. It wasn't quite a voice, but the response I received could not have been clearer. I felt a powerful assurance from God that I would survive the war, and I knew that was what would happen.

When Will got back to Pearl, surprise orders awaited him. He was transferred back to the States to help man a new ship that was being launched. A few months later the

New Orleans was in another savage engagement. To his great sadness, he learned that all the men in his section were killed.

4 Phibbs op. cit. p. 78.
5 Bradley op. cit. pp. 91–2.
6 Bradley op. cit. pp. 92–3, 115, 125.
7 Patton op. cit. p. 104.
8 Boyington op. cit. pp. 371–2.
9 Ibid pp. 372–3.
10 Frankl op. cit. p. 111.

Chapter 17

The Cure of Love:
What the World's Best Copers
Teach Us About Living Well

In the spring of 1999 the men in my two older combat vet groups were struggling with a sharp increase in insomnia, nightmares, irritability and intrusive thoughts of their wars. The cause was the conflict in the Balkans, centered on Kosovo. Every TV channel showed streams of refugees, reported tales of senseless and brutal killings, and talked of "ethnic cleansing." In my WWII vet's minds Milosevic was behaving like Hitler, while his target, the Muslim Kosovars, represented the Jews, Poles, Gypsies and other targets of the Nazi death camps of WWII. It was very difficult to get them to talk about anything therapeutic in group. We kept getting drawn into heated and counter-therapeutic political discussions.

The two groups together totaled 21 men at that time. Of that number, 16 were WWII combat vets, two fought in Korea only, and three others served during Korea and Vietnam. All were 65 years old or older. They were a deep reservoir of experience and knowledge. All had experienced at least several months of continuous combat. Some had spent many years in war zones. Three had survived being POWs. The majority had been decorated for bravery or received Purple Hearts, several both, and some multiple times. They had seen every type of combat on land, sea or air. Many had struggled with alcohol abuse at one time in their lives. Despite this, only one had broken down in combat (after three of his closest friends and most respected leaders were killed the same day), and he had subsequently returned to active duty. All had lived useful and productive lives after their wars.

Hoping to get us doing something therapeutic again, I went to the chalkboard and challenged the men to make a list of the things in their lives that had helped them the most to cope with their war experiences and trauma. They produced a list of eleven items. We worked on the list successfully for months as we explored together why these particular things were therapeutic.

I put things down on the chalkboard chronologically as they brought them up, not necessarily in order of importance. After several sessions spent developing the list and clarifying what each item meant, I had the list typed and copied and asked the men to silently rate the importance of the items for them by putting a one next to the most important item, a two next to the second most important item, and so on. For ease and simplicity I had them just rate the top five of the eleven items one to five in importance. Thus each man left six items unrated.

This is the list of the 11 major therapeutic factors they produced. Behind each item I have listed the number of times the men rated it number one, in the top three, and in the top five.

		Times #	Times top 3	Times top 5
1)	Be busy – jobs, work.	5	11	16
2)	Service to others.	2	7	13
3)	Spiritual – prayer, miracles, meditation.	1	13	18
4)	Loving spouse and family.	6	10	13
5)	Relationships with comrades and friends.	0	9	11
6)	Focusing on positive experiences from the war.	0	0	0
7)	Forgiveness of self and others.	3	6	10
8)	Humor.	1	1	5
9)	Medications for sleep, anxiety and depression.	3	4	7
10)	Avoid sensationalism of the news media.	0	2	4
11)	Pets.	0	1	8

Some of the items seemed to group together naturally. Numbers one and two seemed to the men to overlap so much that they liked the idea of combining them as "staying busy doing good." They felt numbers three and seven also went together under the larger category of "spiritual activity."

Finally they put numbers four and five together as "healthy relationships." These we started referring to as "the Big Three."

Thus the Big Three were:

1) Staying busy doing good (originally # 1 Be busy – jobs, work and # 2 Service to others)
2) Spiritual activity (originally # 3 Spiritual – prayer, miracles, meditation and # 7 Forgiveness of self and others)
3) Healthy relationships (originally # 4 Loving spouse and family and # 5 Relationships with comrades and friends)

The Big Three were evenly balanced in importance in the men's minds. If you add up the total number of ratings in the top three for each pair, you get 18 for "staying busy doing good," 19 for "spiritual activity," and 19 for "healthy relationships." The majority of men rated three of the original six items that combined into "the big three" as the top three therapeutic factors over the course of their lives. The only real point of contention was whether or not number 11, "pets," should be combined with numbers four and five in the "healthy relationships" category! In the end they decided to leave it separate.

One point the men often made was that at different times in their lives, different things had been the most important or most therapeutic. At one time the influence of friends or spouse may have helped the most; another time spiritual activities may have been preeminent; and in another period work or medication made the biggest positive difference for them. When they made their ratings, some say they marked things down according to what was important now; others tried to rate these items for their importance over a whole lifetime.

This list confirmed for me what I felt I had already learned from these men. It sums up and reinforces much of what I have already written in this book. It is also a blueprint for anyone hoping to live a healthy, good life. We all find meaning and purpose in life through productive work, useful service, spiritual exploration and connection, and loving relationships. A rich and abundant life is blessed with all these things. We cannot enjoy any significant happiness without at least some of them.

These items warrant more exploration. Notice first and foremost that most have little to do with any type of formal treatment. The men have led lives that are therapeutic in and of themselves. As in many cases we have already discussed, these men treat themselves in a variety of successful ways. It is analogous to a principle of medical treatment attributed to the ancient Greek physician, Hippocrates: "Do no harm." Following the adage to "do no harm" can be a successful therapeutic strategy for cautious, patient physicians. Humans often heal on their own if we leave them room and opportunity to do so. Nonetheless, as therapists we can foster greater and more complete recovery by getting our patients to seek out and take full advantage of the natural social and spiritual forces of healing all around us.

Staying busy doing good (# 1 and # 2) is a healing principle in the lives of every one of these men. As I discussed in Chapter 3, all of those men returned from the war with symptoms of PTSD. All forced themselves to re-engage in life. They found work, returned to school and started families. As they positively focused on the here and now in productive ways, their nightmares, intrusive thoughts and hyper-alertness began to abate.

Others who continued to use alcohol remained more symptomatic. Some of those, like Doug, struggled for decades with drinking and did not really improve dramatically until they permanently sobered up.

The majority of the 21 men never sought any formal treatment until after they retired. With time on their hands, they had a return of symptoms and sought help from the VA. Many came for medical care initially, but attentive physicians and nurses picked up on their war-related symptoms and successfully referred them to our care. Classic examples are JR (8th Air Force survivor – see Chapter 2) and Sam (*Indianapolis* survivor – see Chapter 3). Both were very busy with their careers and families. Neither sought any treatment until after they became "empty nesters" and retired from work. Now both have returned to active volunteer work to fill that void. Two other men, a plumber and a lumberman, who are now single with less family support, say they will never retire. I support them in this. They need continued activity and involvement to counteract the lack of family support and connection currently in their lives.

Many veterans just flat out tell me, "My wife made the difference" (item # 4). Larry notes his wife finally got him to address and conquer his drinking. Doug's wife is now ill. He says, "She stuck by me through so much; now it's my turn to support her." Mark was doing fine until his wife was killed in a car accident. Then all his post-war symptoms flooded back and he was referred to our care. Children, grandchildren and great-grandchildren continue to add companionship and purpose to life.

The therapeutic influence of comrades and friends has been a constant healing force for almost all (item # 5). Reunions, phone calls, letters and cards have kept them in touch and helped them cope. The groups have been going for so long now that the men involved have formed deep bonds with each other. They support one another in sickness – visiting each other in the hospital. They advocate for each other in the VA system. They have lunch together. They give each other rides to the hospital for medical and therapy appointments. They mourn together when a group member dies in a way they could not mourn during combat. They are now able to say a full good-bye and properly bury their dead. They welcome new men into group when a new vet agrees to "try a little therapy." However, one 1st Marine Division survivor of Guadalcanal, with little family support and limited friendships, still vows that his dog is his most therapeutic friend (item # 11).

Spiritual activity continues to play an important role in the veterans' lives (items # 3 and # 7), just as it has all along for most of them. Some pray every day, claiming that they would not have the strength to face their current health and emotional challenges if they didn't. They talk of receiving comfort and guidance. One recently told me of praying for guidance about what to do with his spouse, who was refusing to get some medical help he knew she needed:

> After praying I had a different thought come into my head about how to approach her. I had never tried it before, and things were getting serious. I followed this bit of inspiration and it worked! I felt God had guided me when everything else I had tried had failed.

Some of the men are involved in active religious fellowships that provide them with opportunities for service and healthy social outlets. Some tell me they pray for me, that I'll continue helping others as I have helped them.

Many continue to pray for peace and forgiveness. They benefit from a deep faith in an afterlife where all wounds will be healed and long-dead enemies will have a chance to meet and reconcile. George (Chapter 4), who led guerilla forces in the Philippines and defeated the Japanese on many occasions by being just as merciless as they were, had this type of faith. We discussed it many times in the last three months of his life as he was dying of cancer at our VA hospital. His faith in a loving God, a reunion with his deceased wife and reconciliation in the afterlife with departed enemies gave him hope and peace.

All of these men are cautious about what they subject themselves to from the media (item # 10). They have learned by sad experience that constant visual and aural exposure to violent stimuli activates and maintains their traumatic symptoms. If they want to have a chance of sleeping, they cannot partake of typical Hollywood "R rated for violence" fare.

Because of a selection bias (I am a psychiatrist, so men are referred to me who others think might need meds.), most of the men I see benefit from medications for sleep, depression, or anxiety disorders (item # 9). For some, medications have resulted in significant improvements in their lives, with a marked decrease in symptoms and minimal side effects.

Gene's experiences in WWII and afterward illustrate almost everything my vets have taught me about war and recovery from war. He grew up dirt poor as his family tried to scratch out a living in Oklahoma before WWII. He joined the Marine Corps the day after Pearl Harbor. He went through basic training and then, because of his aptitude as a soldier, received advanced infantry training and graduated from the Marine Scout and Sniper School at Camp Elliot, California. He participated in the Guadalcanal campaign, which started in August 1942 with the invasion of Tulagi, a small island across Iron Bottom Sound from Guadalcanal. In the sharp fighting on Tulagi he was wounded in the hand. In October 1942 his unit was transferred to Guadalcanal and fought there until the end of January 1943. He relates his story as follows:

> It was intense combat under miserable conditions. We never had enough to eat. We lived off the food and rice that was captured from the Japanese when we first invaded and they hastily withdrew into the jungle. The Japanese were even worse off. Sometimes they ate only insects and the hearts of palm they hacked out of the local trees. I caught malaria but never stopped doing my job. I would go on long patrols two or three times a week as first scout. I should never have survived Guadalcanal. I lived through as many close scrapes as a man could. My number was way overdue.
>
> Initially I didn't hate the Japanese, and though I killed many – that was my job as a sniper – I never did it with hate. I was different in that respect from many of the men. On one patrol a Japanese tried to surrender to us. He was naked except for a loincloth. As he neared us, he reached for something in his loincloth. Everyone in the patrol opened up on him but me. He was chewed to pieces. When we searched him, we found that he was just pulling out a can of fish. I was there several times when Marines shot Japanese prisoners. I couldn't do that, even though I saw the Japanese do horrible things to us, including cutting off Marines' heads and putting them on stakes as a warning that they would do the same to us if we kept fighting. On January 13, 1943, that changed for me. On that day the Japanese killed nine of the twelve men in my squad. Men I loved.

At this point Gene cannot keep talking. He never can when he gets to that day. Tears and pain seem to take over, but there is also shame. He tells me little bits and pieces:

I let hate take over. I used a BAR [Browning automatic rifle] that day to kill many Japanese trapped in bunkers. I fired ten to 15 clips into them as fast as I could. They were like animals trapped in a pen – running and scared; there was no escape. I just kept killing them and I didn't care.

He can't say more about it. Maybe we will eventually be able to explore what happened that day, but not so far. Some parts of a man's story are much harder to share than others. He continues:

We left Guadalcanal for New Zealand January 30, 1943. We rested and trained there until the invasion of Tarawa at the end of 1943. In New Zealand the last two survivors from my original squad were killed in a live fire training exercise when a mortar round fell short. I nearly went crazy with grief and rage. Four other men had to restrain me. I wanted to get at the mortarmen. I don't know what I might have done. It wasn't their fault, though. They were probably defective rounds. I know it must have been bad for them.

The killing at Tarawa exceeded anything I had ever experienced. We were stuck between the ocean and the sea wall. I was an outstanding shot. I got in position on a small pier where the Japanese had to expose themselves to get at me. I had two bandoleers of M-1 ammo, plus several other clips. I used it all as the Japanese kept trying to kill me. Two other marksmen were next to me. They were finally killed, and I used their ammo. At that time it was like at the end of Guadalcanal. I didn't mind the killing. I still had hate left over. There was so much death. Bodies and pieces of bodies were everywhere. The sea had changed color to red. Out of ammo finally, I had to move to find some more and to form up with the rest of my unit. I had several wounds, but none that serious. I crawled around the pier and sea wall until I found the rest of my unit and got more ammo. I was trying to get into a good firing position when my left arm was nearly blown off. A large piece of bone between my shoulder and elbow was gone. The arm was just hanging by skin and muscle. I draped it across my shoulder so it wouldn't tear off completely, but I soon passed out from loss of blood. The other Marines thought I was dead. My younger brother even wrote my mom and told her I was killed. Someone covered me with a poncho. I think I woke up because it got so hot under the poncho. There was another Marine next to me who was wounded in the face and couldn't see. I was too weak to get up or walk, but he said if I would guide him he would carry me to the aid station. When we got there our doc refused to let them give me plasma, saying we needed to save what little we had for those who might live. But I refused to die. With me serving as his eyes, my blind buddy eventually carried me to an evacuation landing craft and we were both transported to the hospital ship.

Two important things happened at Tarawa. First, I had always prayed for protection. Now I had proof God was there, because no one else could have gotten me through that piece of hell and saved me so many times. Second, my hate for the Japanese disappeared. I don't know how it happened. I realized in the middle of the killing that I was praying the war would just end. I didn't care any longer who won. I just wanted the killing to stop. I felt sorry again for the men I was killing, just like I had at the beginning. I had shot so many Japanese. I didn't blame them for shooting me.

Gene was evacuated to Hawaii and the Oakland Naval Hospital. He went through many surgeries. Miraculously, his arm was successfully reattached. "I was told that although two inches of bone was gone, that the radial nerve somehow was intact. It seemed like another miracle to me." He spent the rest of the war recovering from his wounds. "I wanted to stay on in the Marine Corps, but my commanding officer said I wasn't fit for duty. My left arm was just too weak at that time."

Before the end of the war Gene married his high school sweetheart. He had little education but was smart and worked hard. He developed a milk delivery business that by 1968 was worth several million dollars. He continues the story of his post war years:

The killing and nightmares continued to bother me. I had nightmares every night and was constantly trying to get thoughts of the war out of my head. I kept drinking after the war to sleep and not think about the war. The drinking was ruining my marriage. My wife was the sweetest person. You couldn't ask for a better woman, but I couldn't stop drinking. Finally she left and took the three kids with her. I gave her all the property at the divorce. I kept drinking and working, but those were some of my darkest days. I didn't even want to live. In 1971 I met Mary. She was trying to raise two kids on her own. I fell in love again, and the love she and her kids had for me was like a lifeline. It saved me.

    I cut back on the drinking but never stopped. By 1974 the drinking was threatening my second marriage. It was even worse, though, because I was starting to be abusive. I had never done that before. I was getting out of control. I was scared. In desperation I prayed to God and told Him, "I know you can take this desire to drink away from me," and He did! I took a drink twice more a few months later but got physically ill each time. I think God was warning me not to touch the stuff ever again, and since then I never have. After this the nightmares finally began easing up. Before praying for help to stop drinking, I had only thanked God in my prayers since the war. I felt God had given me so much during the war that I couldn't ask for more. But that is wrong. You need to ask Him for everything. My whole life is centered on God now. My wife and I pray together. God helped me with the guilt over killing. I had to do the killing for my country and the Marines I served with. I have no hate for the Japanese. They fought hard just like the Marines. It still bothers me that for a time I killed with hate in my heart, but God has helped even with that. I am grateful to be alive.

Gene struggled with guilt about the killing until he felt God finally helped him stop drinking. He has prayed about and pondered the killing since the war. He did what he had to do. He can now leave the judgments to others, but he feels he can face God and be accepted by Him.

He feels being alive is a miracle and a joy. He loves to fish and teach children to fish. He shares his modest means with others in need. He leads a simple, happy life. The nightmares still occur weekly. He is resigned to taking them to his grave. Someday I hope we can talk through what happened on January 13, 1943. Right now the emotions are too raw to allow a full sharing and exploration. Maybe he is right, though, and it should not be discussed. A man like Gene has to decide when and if it is right to share his horror.

Gene tasted hate at Guadalcanal and Tarawa, but gave it up through the help of his God. Several years after the war Gene's nephew married a Japanese woman. His brother never would talk to her, but Gene welcomed her into the family immediately and they have remained close friends. He had his heart broken by violent war-deaths and divorce. He was trapped by his addiction and the constant memories of war. The reciprocal love of a good woman and her children was a "lifeline" that revived his desire to live and restored meaning to his life. When his second marriage and family were also threatened by his war-related symptoms and his drinking, a desperate plea for divine help was answered in what he sees as a miraculous way. He achieved sobriety. When I look into his face and eyes, I see joy and energy. He has now built a network of love in his life that has healed his heart and given him the hope of a loving and full redemption from the hell of war.

I argued in Chapter 2 that one of the ironies of war is that love is needed to make war possible. Without love for their comrades, most men could not continue to wage war. Combatants without the love that binds them to their fellows more readily succumb to cowardice and a sensible desire for safety, and they flee the battlefield. Combatants with deep love and loyalty to one another find the strength to overcome their fear of death and prevail as a team on the battlefield.[1,2]

Though love makes extended combat possible for most men, deep love of fellow combatants also creates some of the greatest pain from war – as beloved comrades are killed and the survivors suffer profound heartbreak.

But to continue loving is also the cure for war's emotional and spiritual trauma. The important items discussed in this chapter are all facets of love. The most successful post-war combatants surround themselves in a network of love. The reciprocal love of spouse, family, comrades, and friends sustains the heart and soul as it heals. Productive work and service are acts of love. Men's private spiritual devotions and prayers help them feel connected to and blessed by a Divine love. Acting on love and being truthful, merciful and forgiving after their wars generate hope in the combatants' hearts that reconciliation and peace are possible.

In a beautiful article written in 1960, entitled "On the Therapeutic Action of Psycho-analysis," Hans Loewald argues that in the end successful therapy "is in essence a cure through love."[3] My veterans have taught me this in my work with them. Love makes it possible for good men to wage war and survive. It also provides the path out of hell and the balm needed to heal war's wounds.

Notes

1   Sledge op. cit. p. 323. See the next to last paragraph for Sledge's own thoughts on the importance of love amongst fellow combatants.
2   Rickenbacker, Capt. Eddie V., *Fighting the Flying Circus*, pp. 320–1. See Rickenbacker's last two sentences for his own thoughts on the deep ties that bind fellow combatants together.
3   Loewald, Hans, "On the Therapeutic Action of Psychoanalysis", *Int. J. Psychoanal*, Jan–Feb; 41:16–33 p. 32.

Bibliography

This is a listing of the biographies, diaries, memoirs, studies of history and articles used in preparing this book. The vast majority of the books are autobiographical accounts written by the soldiers themselves, or war histories that I have found useful in understanding the context of war when treating veterans. I have cited current popular editions and paperbacks where possible as these are more readily available to the therapists, soldiers and general public who might want to read further. In cases where I list two editions, the citations I have used come from the more popular second listing.

Allen, Thomas B. and Norman Polmar, *Code-Name Downfall: The Secret Plan To Invade Japan And Why Truman Dropped The Bomb*, New York: Simon & Schuster, 1995.

Ambrose, Stephen E., *Band of Brothers*, New York: Simon & Schuster, 1992.

Ambrose, Stephen E., *D-Day: June 6, 1944: The Climactic Battle of World War II*, New York: Simon & Schuster, 1994.

Ambrose, Stephen E., *Citizen Soldiers*, New York: Simon & Schuster, 1997.

Anderson, Col. Clarence E. "Bud" with Joseph P. Hamelin, *To Fly And Fight*, New York: St. Martin, 1990. Bantam, 1991.

Ankrum, Homer R., *Dogfaces Who Smiled Through Tears*, Lake Mills, Iowa: Graphic Publishing, 1987.

Balkoski, Joseph, *Beyond The Beachhead*, Harrisburg, Pennsylvania: Stackpole Books, 1989. New York: Dell, 1992.

Boyington, Gregory "Pappy", *Baa Baa Black Sheep*, New York: Putnam, 1958. Bantam, 1977.

Bradley, James with Ron Powers, *Flags of Our Fathers*, New York: Bantam, 2000.

Brokaw, Tom, *The Greatest Generation*, New York: Random House, 1998.

Brickhill, Paul, *Reach for the Sky*, New York: Ballantine, 1954.

Chesley, Capt. Larry, *Seven Years In Hanoi*, Salt Lake City, Utah: Bookcraft, 1973.

Clewell, Richard D. "Moral Dimensions in Treating Combat Veterans with Posttraumatic Stress Disorder", *Bulletin of the Menninger Clinic*, 51(1), January, 114–30, 1986.

Collins, Brig. Gen. James L. and Lt. Col. Eddy Bauer, *The Marshall Cavendish Illustrated Encyclopedia of World War II*, New York: Marshall Cavendish Corporation, 1972.

Cortesi, Lawrence, *Gateway To Victory*, New York: Zebra Books, 1984.

Craig, William, *The Fall of Japan*, New York: Penguin Books, 1967.

Davis, Russell, *Marine at War*, New York: Scholastic Book Services, 1961.

Daws, Gavan, *Prisoners of the Japanese*, New York: Morrow, 1994.

Dissette, Edward and H.C. Adamson, *Guerrilla Submarines*, New York: Ballantine, 1972.

Dupuy, Trevor Nevitt, *The Military History of World War II: Vols. 1–17*, New York: Franklin Watts, Inc, 1962.

Ethell, Jeffrey and Alfred Price, *One Day In a Long War*, New York: Random House, 1989.

Ethell, Jeffrey and Alfred Price, *Target Berlin*, London: Jane's Publishing, 1981, Arms and Armor Press, 1989.

Fahey, James J., *Pacific War Diary*, New York: Avon Books, 1963.

FitzPatrick, Bernard T. with John A. Sweetser III, *The Hike into the Sun*, Jefferson, North Carolina: McFarland & Company, 1993.

Forester, C.S., *Sink the Bismarck!*, New York: Curtis Publishing, 1958. Bantam, 1959.

Forrester, Larry, *Fly for Your Life*, New York: Frederick Muller Ltd., 1956. Bantam, 1978.

Frankl, Victor, *Man's Search for Meaning*, Boston: Beacon Press, 1946 & 1959, New York: Washington Square Press, 1985.

Fuchida, Mitsuo and Masatake Okumiya, *Midway: The Battle that Doomed Japan*, Annapolis, Maryland: U.S Naval Institute, 1955. New York: Ballantine, 1958.

Galantin, Admiral I.J., *Take Her Deep!*, New York: Pocket Books, 1987.

Gavan, Gen. James M., *On To Berlin*, New York: Viking, 1978. Bantam, 1979.

Goldstein, Donald M., Katherine V. Dillon and J. Michael Wenger, *Pearl Harbor: The Original Photographs*, Washington: Brassey's (US), Inc, 1991.

Grinker, Roy R. and John P. Spiegel, *War Neuroses*, Philadelphia: Blakiston, 1945.

Grossman, Lt. Col. Dave, *On Killing*, New York: Little, Brown and Company, 1995, 1996.

Harkins, Philip, *Blackburn's Headhunters*, New York: W.W. Norton and Company, 1955.

Hastings, Major Donald W., Captain David G. Wright, and Captain Bernard C. Glueck, *Psychiatric Experiences of the Eighth Air Force, First Year of Combat (July 4, 1942-July 4, 1943)*, Prepared and Distributed for The Air Surgeon Army Air Forces by the Josiah Macy, Jr. Foundation: New York 21, NY 1943.

Hechler, Ken, *The Bridge at Remagen*, New York: Ballantine, 1957.

Heiferman, Ronald, *World War II*, New York: Octopus Books, 1973.

Hendin, Herbert, M.D. and Ann Pollinger Haas, Ph.D. "Combat Adaptations of Vietnam Veterans Without Posttraumatic Stress Disorders", *American Journal of Psychiatry*, 141(8), August, 956–60, 1984.

Hersey, John, *Of Men and War*, New York: Scholastic Inc. 1963, 1991.

Hiroshima-Nagasaki Publishing Committee, *Hiroshima-Nagasaki: A Pictorial Record of the Atomic Destruction*, Japan: 1978.

Hoyt, Edwin P., *The Battle of Leyte Gulf*, New York: David McKay Company, 1972. Jove, 1983.

Hoyt, Edwin P., *Bowfin*, New York: Van Nostrand Reinhold Company, 1983. Avon Books, 1984.

Hoyt, Edwin P., *The Destroyer Killer*, New York: Pocket Books, 1989.

Hunt, Ray C. and Bernard Norling, *Behind Japanese Lines*, New York: The University Press of Kentucky, 1986. Pocket Books, 1988.

Hynes, Samuel, *Flights of Passage*, New York: Pocket Books, 1988.

Jablonski, Edward, *Airwar* (two volumes in one: *Outraged Skies* and *Wings Of Fire*). Garden City, New York: Doubleday & Company, 1971.

Jacobs, Bruce, *Heroes of the Army*, New York: W.W. Norton and Company, 1956. Berkley, 1960, 1963.

Johnson, Franklyn A., *One More Hill*, New York: Bantam, 1983.

Leinbaugh, Harold and John Campbell, *The Men of Company K*, New York: Bantam, 1985.

Levi, Primo, *Survival in Auschwitz*, New York: Collier Books, 1986.

Loewald, Hans W. "On the Therapeutic Action of Psychoanalysis", *International Journal of Psychoanalysis*, 41, January–February (1960), pp. 16–33.

Lopez, Donald S., *Into the Teeth of the Tiger*, New York: Bantam, 1986.

Lord, Walter, *Incredible Victory*, New York: Harper & Row, 1967. Pocket Books, 1968.

Lorenz, Conrad, *On Aggression*, New York: Harcourt, Brace & World (English Ed.), 1966. Bantam, 1967.

MacDonald, Charles B., *The Battle of the Huertgen Forest*, New York: J.B. Lippincott, 1963. Jove, 1983.

MacDonald, Charles B., *Company Commander*, New York: US Army, 1947. Bantam, 1978.

Mahedy, William P., *Out of the Night*, New York: Ballantine, 1986.

Manchester, William, *Good-bye Darkness*, New York: Dell, 1979.

Marshall, S.L.A., *Pork Chop Hill*, New York: William Morrow and Company, 1956. Jove, 1986.

Mayo, Lida, *Bloody Buna*, New York: Doubleday, 1974. Playboy Press, 1979.

Michener, James, *The Bridge at Andau*, Greenwich, Connecticut: Fawcett Publications, Inc. 1957.

Miller, John Grider, *The Bridge at Dong Ha*, Annapolis, Maryland: US Naval Institute Press, 1989.

Monks, John P., *College Men at War*, Boston: American Academy of Arts and Sciences, Memoirs, Vol. 24, 1957.

Moore, Lt. Gen. Harold G. and Joseph L. Galloway, *We Were Soldiers Once ... and Young*, New York: Random House, 1992.

Morison, Samuel Eliot, *History of U.S. Naval Operations in World War II*, 15 vols, Boston: Little, Brown and Company: 1947–62.

Morison, Samuel Eliot, *John Paul Jones*, New York: Little, Brown and Company, 1959. Time-Life Books, 1964.

Murphy, Audie, *To Hell and Back*, New York: Holt, Rinehart and Winston, 1949. Bantam, 1979.

O'Donnell, Patrick K., *Beyond Valor*, New York: The Free Press, 2001.

O'Kane, Richard H., *Clear The Bridge*, New York: Rand McNally, 1977. Bantam, 1981.

Overy, Richard, *Why the Allies Won*, New York: W.W. Norton & Company, 1995.

Patton, George S. Jr., *War as I Knew It*, New York: Houghton Mifflin, 1947. Bantam, 1980.

Peterson, Richard, PhD., *Healing the Child Warrior*, Cardiff by the Sea, California: Consultors Inc. 1992.

Phibbs, Brendan, *The Other Side of Time*, New York: Little, Brown and Company, 1987. Pocket Books, 1989.

Pyle, Ernie, *Here is Your War*, New York: Lancer Books, 1943.

Rankin, Hugh F., *Francis Marion: The Swamp Fox*, New York: Thomas Y. Crowell Company, 1973.

Rawnsley, C.F. and Robert Wright, *Night Fighter*, New York: Ballantine, 1957, 1967.

Rhodes, Anthony, *Propaganda: The Art of Persuasion in World War II*, New York: Chelsea House, 1976.

Rickenbacker, Capt. Eddie V., *Fighting the Flying Circus*, New York: Avon Books, 1967, First copyright 1919.

Roscoe, Theodore, *Pig Boats*, New York: US Naval Institute, 1949. Bantam, 1958.

Schwarzkopf, General Norman H. with Peter Petre, *It Doesn't Take a Hero*, New York: Bantam, 1992.

Scott, Col. Robert L., *God is my Co-Pilot*, New York: Ballantine, 1943.

Sides, Hampton, *Ghost Soldiers*, New York: Doubleday, 2001.

Sledge, E.B., *With the Old Breed at Peleliu and Okinawa*, New York: Bantam, 1983.

Smith, S.E., editor, *The United States Marine Corps in World War II*, New York: Random House, 1969.

Sontag, Sherry and Christopher Drew with Annette Lawrence Drew, *Blind Man's Bluff*, New York: HarperCollins, 1998. Perennial, 2000.

Stafford, Cmdr. Edward P., *The Big E*, New York: Random House, 1962. Ballantine, 1974.

Steinberg, Rafael, *Island Fighting*, Alexandria, VA: WWII Time-Life Books, 1978.

Sterling, Forest J., *Wake of the Wahoo*, New York: Popular Library, 1960.

Thomas, Gordon and Max Morgan Witts, *Enola Gay*, New York: Pocket Books, 1977.

Toland, John, *Battle: The Story of the Bulge*, New York: Random House, 1959.

Toland, John, *In Mortal Combat*, New York: Morrow, 1991.

Toland, John, *The Rising Sun*, New York: Random House, 1970. Bantam, 1971.

Tregaskis, Richard, *Guadalcanal Diary*, Garden City, NY: Blue Ribbon Books, 1943.

Volckmann, R.W., *We Remained*, New York: W.W. Norton and Company, 1954.

Waller, Willard, *The Veteran Comes Back*, New York: The Dryden Press, 1944.

Wilcox, Hazel with Ruth Wheeler, *Angels Over Manila*, Mountain View, California: Pacific Press, 1980.

Wilson, George, *If You Survive*, New York: Ivy Books, 1987.

Wolfert, Ira, *American Guerilla In the Philippines*, New York: Simon & Schuster, 1945. Bantam, 1980.

Index

Many of the veteran patients in this book are referred to only by a first name or nickname. In the index only that same first name or nickname is referenced.

3 5898 00167 1532

LINEBERGER
MEMORIAL LIBRARY
LUTHERAN THEOLOGICAL
SOUTHERN SEMINARY
COLUMBIA, SOUTH CAROLINA 29203

DEMCO